"A must-read for anyone who treats adult ch
(ACEIPs). Lindsay C. Gibson's clinician's guide
work tailored for the unique obstacles faced by those who grew up with an emotionally
immature attachment figure. Gibson's expertise and empathy shine through, offering
practitioners the insights and strategies needed to support our ACEIP clients toward
flourishing in self-alignment."

> —**Simona Vivi H**, founder of the Center for Remothering and of
> www.remothering.org

"Lindsay C. Gibson has done it again! Whether you are a seasoned clinician or an early
practitioner, this book will provide you with powerful strategies for helping ACEIPs. Her
practical instructions provide a road map for deep emotional repair work. I love this work
and strongly recommend it for all clinicians under my supervision."

> —**Anna Baranowsky, PhD, CPsych**, clinical director at Bear Psychology,
> CEO and founder of the Traumatology Institute and Trauma Practice, and
> author of *Trauma Practice*

"Masterful at helping clinicians understand ACEIPs and their emotionally immature
parents (EIPs), this book offers background information on ACEIPs and EIPs, theoretical
knowledge, important techniques, vignettes, and lists of ideas critical to working with
ACEIPs. Containing an encyclopedic amount of knowledge, the book will deepen and
strengthen your work with ACEIPs, and you will undoubtedly find yourself referring to it
when working with this important population."

> —**Ed Neukrug**, Batten Endowed Chair of Counseling at Old Dominion
> University, fellow of the American Counseling Association (ACA),
> and recent winner of the ACA publications award

"Imagine having a wise, talented psychologist sitting beside you as you learn new skills in
working with ACEIPs. In this book, Lindsay C. Gibson not only provides a guide for this
work, but she also shares potential roadblocks that may occur and suggestions for how to
move through them with illustrations from her own work."

> —**Esther Lerman Freeman, PsyD**, associate professor, retired,
> Oregon Health and Science University

"This book is rich, readable, and practical! Lindsay C. Gibson is among my top ten go-to resources for working deeply with clients. This guide synthesizes current theoretical approaches, offering clinicians valuable treatment steps, empathic strategies, and useful tools for assisting clients to effectively process and grow from their formative experiences. Gibson also strikes the right balance between encouraging support and helpful psycho-education for further developing our clinical selves."

—**Suzan K. Thompson, PhD**, consultant and licensed professional
counselor in private practice in Virginia with more than thirty years
of clinical practice experience

"After reading Lindsay C. Gibson's latest book, I find myself feeling so grateful for her emotionally mature voice in this world. Therapists will find both practical and profound guidance here. Having put language to what for so many ACEIPs has felt like ineffable pain, she has both validated and oriented us to our experiences and guided us out of suffering. This book now teaches therapists how to do the same for clients."

—**Jenny Walters, MA**, licensed marriage and family therapist, and
founder of Highland Park Holistic Psychotherapy in Los Angeles, CA

"In *Treating Adult Children of Emotionally Immature Parents*, Lindsay C. Gibson offers compassionate guidance and practical strategies to help adults heal from the lingering effects of childhood wounds, empowering readers to develop healthier relationships and reclaim their emotional well-being. This insightful book is a vital resource for anyone navigating the complexities of parental influence on adult life."

—**Britt Frank, LSCSW, SEP**, author of *The Science of Stuck* and
The Getting Unstuck Workbook

"This is THE book we have been waiting for, providing a comprehensive framework with practical interventions needed to effectively treat ACEIPs. With a voice of humility, expertise, and authenticity, Gibson provides expert guidance, equipping therapists with skills to support clients in overcoming their past to feel healthy, happy, and whole. An absolute must-read for every clinician."

—**Tiffany Wentz-Root, MA, LMHC, ACS**, corporate resilience and
wellness facilitator, and founder of Resilient Roots

Treating
Adult Children *of*
Emotionally
Immature
Parents

A Clinician's Guide

LINDSAY C. GIBSON, PsyD

New Harbinger Publications, Inc.

Introduction

I've wanted to write this book since I first began training to become a therapist myself. I soaked up ideas from the therapy books I loved, but when it came to applying them, the gap between the instructions I was reading and my inexperience seemed enormous.

My first psychotherapy session felt traumatic. I remember entering the room, holding the door for my first client, sitting down opposite them, and feeling alarmed that my hearing was all but annihilated by the roaring in my ears. I didn't think I was *that* nervous, although I knew I lacked confidence and felt out of my element with this real person in front of me. But my body knew how scared I was. It was screaming that this was a life-threatening situation and I should *run*. However, I was well accustomed to sitting tight and looking calm while panicking inside, so I stayed put and listened—to the roaring in my head.

I've never had that happen since, but it taught me that inexperience can be terrifying. I don't recall now, but I assume that I calmed down and was eventually able to listen to that new client instead of my own anxiety symptom. Later, I wished I had been more emotionally prepared for what felt like being tossed into the deep end of the pool for my first swimming lesson. Surely I didn't have to feel so panicked and unprepared as I launched into my intended field?

Now, with plenty of experience under my belt, I still have moments when I don't know what to do. Everyone does. But the difference now is that I have an array of possible interventions to try, and so no longer feel anxiety due to a sheer lack of knowledge. I'm also sure now that my heart is in the right place, and that at least I'm probably not going to make anybody worse. Now anxiety mostly pops up when I'm unsure how to take us where we need to go—i.e., into something deeper and closer to the root of the problem.

But I don't panic; I just notice when I'm not in the groove, and I readjust. I listen for what my instincts are saying. I connect with my true self and seek attunement with my client so I can sense the true nature of their predicament. Sharing what I have learned about *how* to deepen this attunement is a major goal of this book.

Whatever your level of therapy experience, this book will help you do restorative, transformative work with adult children of emotionally immature parents (ACEIPs). These clients have a special set of issues that this book can help you be aware of and ready for. The biggest problem for a therapist working with these clients is that the adult child of emotionally immature parents (ACEIPs) is so accustomed to hiding their inner world that it can be hard to engage them at a deeper emotional level. Not only do they appear more mature and self-sufficient than they really feel, but they can be such avid students that you may feel tempted to be their teacher or mentor instead of their therapist.

Therapy with such well-behaved clients can reach a point of stagnation, where the client seems to stay on the surface, paddling around in circles and talking about things that don't take you into anything deep or interesting. You might feel bored. You may even feel tempted to end this therapy that has devolved into the client's safe and dutiful reporting of the mundane and superficial. The solution is always to seek these clients' deeper side, and what's most emotionally alive for them in the moment.

Many ACEIPs haven't experienced relationships as places where they can really be themselves. They don't expect people—even therapists—to *really* want to know what they experience in their inner world. Trying to be low maintenance, they adopted a self-protective superficiality with their parents, and now they use it to preserve their relationship with you. Sometimes the hardest part of therapy with ACEIPs is convincing them that you think their need for help is legitimate.

Working with ACEIPs will deepen your sensitivity and emotional awareness toward all your clients because ACEIPs' experiences reflect the common and excruciating conditions of loneliness, conflict with loved ones, and feelings of invalidation. Anyone distressed enough to seek therapy has probably had significant encounters with emotionally immature people (EIPs) in childhood or adulthood.

I believe that whatever effectiveness I have with ACEIPs comes from relating to them at the deepest, most human level I can achieve in each moment. It also seems extremely validating to them that my theory about why they feel the way they do goes right to the heart of their oldest childhood emotional predicaments.

The order of this book's chapters is designed to prepare you to do your best possible work with ACEIPs. The first three chapters, taken together, present the foundational understandings necessary for becoming an effective ACEIP therapist. Chapter 1 explores the nature of ACEIPs and their basic human needs, while chapter 2 supplies an understanding of the characteristics and different types of emotionally immature (EI) parents. The psychological costs to your client of having relationships with EIPs will be revealed in chapter 3, and in chapter 4, you'll have a chance to explore your therapeutic stance and preferred approach to therapy.

Starting in chapter 5, we'll focus on helping your client reverse the impact of EI relationships. Then in chapters 6 through 10, I will share the specific techniques that I've found to be particularly effective for ACEIPs, from personality parts work and deep emotional processing to transforming old emotional learnings. You'll become equipped to help your clients change the underlying protective motivations that created their symptoms. You'll enable them to release the symptom, not just fight it with counteractive measures.

And you'll learn about setting up juxtaposition experiences, based on memory reconsolidation brain research, that can cancel out beliefs that have been in control for years. All this will help your client build confidence in their inner experience and feel healthily entitled to protect themselves with personal boundaries and independent minds.

To get the most out of this book, I recommend you keep a notebook handy for making notes and answering questions and exercises you'll find throughout the book, creating a collection of reflections to which you can refer (and add) to later. Visit http://www.newharbinger.com/53592 to download free tools for this book including client handouts and bonus information on special circumstances you may encounter in your work with ACEIP clients.

As you're reading the early chapters and perhaps itching to get on to the techniques, be assured I don't spend a moment longer than necessary to help you build out a deep understanding of what your ACEIP client is facing. The first half of this manual is designed to foster empathy for your client and to increase your own self-awareness, developments that will make *any* technique you use more effective. Technique works best when it extends from a fully grasped theory, and my aim is to make the theory interesting and useful to you as we tie it to clinical experience.

In this book you'll learn my favorite aspects of several different therapy systems, so you can integrate all the techniques I've found work best with ACEIPs. I believe that the best therapy borrows pieces from all kinds of methodologies, and I urge you to read and study further the approaches herein that you find most interesting. The more you learn and integrate varied theories and techniques, the more resources and depth you will bring to your psychotherapy sessions.

Deepening your understanding of ACEIPs' experiences and the impact of EIPs on their lives will make your work with them more interesting and rewarding. Their self-doubts, unmet emotional needs, and relationship struggles are the aftermath of growing up with egocentric people who protect their own interests at the expense of their children's self-worth. Once you grasp what they've been up against, effective therapeutic interventions will come more easily.

One of the most meaningful things you can do for a psychotherapy client is to be an enlightened witness (Miller, 1997) to the enormity of what they're trying to do. In therapy together, you and your ACEIP client will be working to reverse their childhood adaptations of subjugation, inhibition, existential unworthiness, self-inflicted erroneous conclusions, and foundational relationship patterns that took years to form. In other words, the two of you will be attempting nothing less than an emotional, existential, and intellectual overhaul of their basic operating systems. The hope you offer them is not only *I'll help you feel better*, but also, *it's hard, but you can do it.*

This book will show you how to emotionally connect with these clients so you can guide them toward deeper connections with their true self. Perhaps you, too, have experienced the common problem of dealing with people whose demands for attention and control overshadow others' needs and freedom to be themselves. As you accompany them in this process, you may also become more self-aware and sympathetic to your own true self. Through the process of therapy, you and your client both may improve your ability to know, love, and value yourself, and to be present and empowered in your own life.

Perhaps that was the root cause of my roaring ears in that first session with my first client—the fear that my true self wasn't going to be enough for the job. Maybe I thought I somehow had to be more than who I really was before I could be a good therapist. I was terrified that my client would be expecting a maturity I didn't yet have.

ACEIPs face this kind of anxiety all the time, feeling that they have to stretch themselves to meet others' expectations in ways that are unrealistic and exhausting. My biggest problem in that first session was that I couldn't believe I could take the time I needed to get comfortable as a newcomer. I didn't feel I had the right to feel as insecure as I certainly was. So here we are at a foundational lesson for any therapist: you can't be more than who you are. But you can learn to make who you are work for you and your clients. That's what effective therapists do.

You don't need to rise above who you are or the level you're at. The right basics are enough. Just remember that at the core of treating another human being, there is only connecting with empathy and understanding in a nonjudging way, while giving them new perspectives that will lead them toward more enlivened ways of being.

My approach is a restorative therapy because my aim is to restore to a person their birthright and potential as a self-aware individual. As an ACEIP therapist, you'll be helping restart a growth process that stalled and went into hiding when your clients, as children, had to change themselves in order to feel even a small measure of acceptance and love from their parent or caregivers. Together, you'll be restoring their connection to self and their ability to make full use of all their gifts.

As a therapist, you know that psychotherapy is more than a way to make a living. It's a unique expedition into psychological depths that increasingly makes our lives feel more truly our own. Every time we help a person uncover the things they sensed but didn't yet know, we help them retrieve pieces of themselves while we learn more about ourselves as well. I'm about to tell you everything I know about working with ACEIPs. I'm excited for you to go through this process, and I hope you'll let me know how it's going for you.

Chapter 1

Being an ACEIP

Adult children of emotionally immature parents (ACEIPs) face emotional injuries and stifled personal development as a result of interactions with emotionally immature (EI) parents. To help them, we need to understand what happened to them so they can restart the reclamation of their true self. This chapter, and the two that follow, will build your understanding of parental emotional immaturity and how it has shaped your clients.

The Two Kinds of ACEIP

Not all children of EI parents turn out the same. In fact, they tend to polarize into one of two types whose coping styles are so different that nearly everything about how each type of ACEIP moves through the world is as different as can be. I call the two types of ACEIPs *internalizers* and *externalizers* (Gibson, 2015).

Depending on your clinical setting, you might see more of one type than the other. A person who seeks out psychotherapy tends to be an internalizer, while an externalizer is more likely to come to therapy unwillingly, such as through court referrals, rehabilitation programs, or under a relationship or work ultimatum. As you'll see, internalizers are capable of being deeply healed by a therapeutic relationship that helps them to name and understand their struggles. Conversely, externalizers tend to expect *others* to change to make *them* feel better. While I'll discuss the externalizer type here, so that you can recognize their style when you encounter them, treating the *internalizer* type of ACEIP is what this book is about. Beyond this chapter, when I mention ACEIPs without the "externalizer" qualification, I will be referring to the internalizer type.

Internalizer Characteristics

Internalizers are intrinsically motivated by their need to understand things and grow psychologically. So, therapy makes sense to them as an effective and interesting way to get stronger and gain self-mastery. They're already accustomed to thinking about things and seeking insight to solve challenges. Because they instinctively try to understand feelings and motivations, they already speak therapy's language.

Internalizers enjoy learning about relationships and self-improvement. They notice their emotional experiences, and they process them thoroughly. They look beneath the surface and wonder about underlying meanings. They tend to be idealistic, sensitive, and empathic, and often find themselves in the roles of confidant, caretaker, or peacemaker within their families growing up. Many of them have been *parentified* (Minuchin et al., 1967; Boszormenyi-Nagy, 1984), or conscripted as emotional support to an EI parent.

Internalizers usually think before they act and are willing to self-reflect on their possible part in any life problems they're having. They can be honest with themselves about their shortcomings, and they feel like they cope better once they've gotten to the bottom of things.

Internalizers are much more likely to be aware of unpleasant internal states like shame, guilt, and self-doubt, because they can tolerate difficult feelings. They can contain and process internal conflict without the need to reduce uncertainty by jumping to conclusions. This gives them the ability to take the time needed to problem-solve all aspects of a situation. Their objectivity and psychological complexity suggest a more mature level of emotional development.

Internalizer ACEIPs probably start life with neurological capacities that facilitate insight and make it interesting to them. Perhaps they come into this world with more innate perceptiveness and sensitivity (Conradt et al., 2013), noticing everything and trying to understand and integrate their experiences into their view of the world. These traits may help explain why they seem more self-reliant and sensible than their less emotionally mature siblings.

However, in their idealism and desire to help others, internalizers can overlook what *they* need to thrive. They may worry about questions of loyalty and moral duty to the point where they neglect their own well-being and boundaries. Many internalizers have steered their life by feelings of guilt and obligation, resulting in trouble setting limits with needy or domineering people. They can also lack a sense of healthy entitlement and self-worth sufficient to protect their interests, and they are often overly self-sacrificing, especially when it comes to family. By caring too much about other people's expectations, they can narrow their lives in ways that constrict their autonomy, growth, and individuation.

Externalizer Characteristics

Externalizer ACEIPs see the world in a more immediate, egocentric way than internalizers do. They're generally oriented toward immediate gratification and blame others when things don't go well in their lives, rather than considering their own role. In therapy, they want quick results; if steered toward self-analysis and slow-but-sure progress, they are likely to lose interest fast. Insight for its own sake doesn't interest them. They may be wary of a therapist's suggestions or demanding in the therapeutic relationship.

Emotional immaturity and externalizing are two sides of the same coin. EIPs are externalizers who oversimplify or deny complex realities, are intolerant of differences, hyperfocus on pet issues, and distort reality according to their preoccupations. They don't self-reflect, and they reject accountability to avoid shame and low self-esteem. They can't tolerate anxiety or discomfort for long, and quickly accuse others of causing their problems. They tend to quickly form rigid, black-and-white judgments in whatever way makes them feel best about themselves.

Externalizers think *others* should change, not them, and so are unlikely to seek psychotherapy unless it appears to be the lesser of two evils—for instance, placating an upset partner or complying with a court order. Because most are not internally motivated to change, they often expect the therapist to "fix" them—or, more likely, to fix their circumstances.

Externalizers ignore other people's viewpoints. To them, their problems exist because they've been treated unfairly, and someone should step in to make it up to them. Even a therapist who goes along with this victimized stance will be discounted as soon as they suggest something the externalizer doesn't like. Chronically dissatisfied, externalizers quickly forget the last thing you did for them. They have a low tolerance for stress and often act as though they believe others have a moral obligation to appease them.

If externalizers sound emotionally immature, it's because they are. And using externalizing coping mechanisms ensures continuing emotional immaturity. Since externalizers don't notice or weigh their effect on others, they don't tend to wonder if they should change their own behavior. Yet the behaviors that flow from their immature coping style will keep getting them in trouble and alienating others.

When Internalizers Attach to Externalizers

An internalizing person with EI parents can be drawn to externalizers, partly because their style feels familiar, but also because their seemingly carefree and even impulsive manner can feel freeing to a conscientious internalizer. But later, when the internalizer begins to hold the externalizer accountable for what they do and say, the externalizer may become defensive and critical in ways that cause the internalizer to doubt themselves.

The internalizer is all too ready to question their own behavior and reactions. Their instinct is to take responsibility when the externalizer starts to complain. The internalizer ends up doing all the *emotional work* (Fraad, 2008) in a relationship with an externalizer, seeking harmony by trying to change themselves and their own behavior. Their coping styles mesh in a way: the internalizer gains a sense of control by trying to improve themselves, and the externalizer feels relieved as soon as they blame someone else. The results demoralize the internalizer, who just can't believe that the externalizer isn't interested in trying as hard as they are. But they keep trying to connect, while the externalizer keeps projecting the blame for their own failures in the relationship.

Can Externalizers Change?

Externalizers change only if they begin to realize they might be playing a role in some of their hardships—something they don't often have the maturity or wisdom to see. Their default is to defend their point of view at all costs and to get others to fall in line with their wishes. Since they tend to use a lot of projection and denial in their assessment of situations, it's hard for a therapist to feel confident they're getting a reasonably accurate picture of the externalizer's life.

Since externalizers are much less likely than internalizers to seek out psychotherapy, your self-referred ACEIP clients will usually be internalizers. You may still see externalizers, either individually or in couples work, but as mentioned, they tend to seek therapy because someone is forcing them to. They may benefit from therapy when externally referred, but it can take a lot of time and work to help an externalizer step back and examine their own reactions and behaviors and their effects on other people.

Emotional Maturity on a Continuum

It can help to think of emotional maturity as being on a continuum, with a person's relative immaturity determined by their tendencies toward egocentrism and rigidity of thought. A more adequately mature adult tends to stay within a certain range that is characterized by a capacity for empathy, self-reflection, and deep connection. However, whether mostly mature or immature, a person's level of emotional maturity might improve or degrade slightly under variable life circumstances—showing more immature reactions under stress or rising to more mature functioning when stress is low and things are going their way, for a time at least.

Under intense stress, even internalizers may temporarily *regress* and react immaturely, like externalizers. This is true for most of us. None of us is at our best when we're fatigued, ill, or stressed. However, internalizers are more likely to resume mature functioning once they regain their balance or the stress eases, whereas externalizers usually don't.

Externalizers are especially likely to show more reactivity and impulsivity under stress, especially when they feel threatened or when their relationships demand more emotional intimacy. But when highly motivated to get something they want, externalizers can temporarily *stretch* themselves to behave more maturely and show more empathy. When feeling good and trying to impress, they can seem much more considerate and self-reflective, but they won't be able to maintain this over the long haul.

Same Family, Different Capabilities

It can be mystifying how different two children of the same parents can be in their level of emotional maturity. Many families with at least one highly capable and responsible adult child have others who seem to struggle with adult life. I propose three common reasons for this disparity: differences in innate sensitivity; different family roles, including parentification; and the presence of supportive relationships outside the family.

Innate Sensitivity

A more emotionally mature child in a family—usually an internalizer—may have greater than average levels of innate sensitivity and perceptiveness. Perhaps they're born with neurological abilities that make them more alert and responsive to their environment than other children (Conradt et al., 2013). Their sensitivity to others' emotional expressions may allow them to "do more with a little"—to notice and grow from even fleeting moments of responsiveness and attention from their caretakers.

EI parents sometimes do respond to their children with unguarded and genuine attention, however briefly, before their defenses rush in. Being alert to these flashes of attunement, internalizer children may take in more emotional nurturance than a less sensitive and aware child. Perhaps the internalizer experiences more connection because they notice it faster, before it disappears.

Parentification and Family Role

Some children come to be relied on by a parent to be a kind of third parent or co-parent (Minuchin et al., 1967; Boszormenyi-Nagy, 1984/2013). This can take the form of either *functional* or *emotional* parentification (Dariotis et al., 2023). For instance, a child is *functionally* parentified when they help with other children, home chores, or other adult responsibilities. The parent trusts—or at least expects—this child to be responsible beyond their years. This responsible family role is not always detrimental as it seems to increase resilience and maturity in some children.

However, when a child is *emotionally* parentified, as a kind of parent, partner, or therapist to the parent—serving as a listener, confidant, or fixer for the parent's emotional distress or need—such a child might be inappropriately privy to their parent's marital complaints, painful childhood memories, or adult problems. The emotional burdening of these emotionally parentified children may result in more psychological issues in adulthood, including depression, than those who were functionally parentified (Dariotis et al., 2023).

Whichever pattern of parentification holds, it's easy to imagine that the EI parent finds it tempting to rely on the internalizer's natural gifts—seeing their sensitive, perceptive child as someone to lean on or to confide in. A sensitive, intellectually gifted child may be especially likely to receive their parents' confidences (Ruf, 2023), especially if the parents lack quality listening and support in their personal lives. These children's precocious comprehension is often irresistible to a lonely parent who doesn't feel they have people they can confide in.

Therapist Tiffany Wentz-Root sees these highest-functioning children in a family as having served as their parent's caretaker. While this is an inappropriate burden for a child, some children nevertheless get the message that they are good thinkers, responsible people, and essential to their parent's equilibrium or the family's stability. These realizations can bring feelings of validation and worthiness. Although being seen as offering valuable caretaking support to the parent can be strengthening to a child's sense of self and feelings of independence, their emotional center is still going unnurtured.

Parentified children are often referred to as "old souls"—wise and calm beyond their years. But they can pay for their precocity by harboring a squishy center of insecurity and loneliness, a wound formed in their earliest unsupported years.

Relationships That Strengthen

Precociously mature children of EI parents could also be seen as *resilient* or as turning out better than one might expect given their background. Studies on resilience (Werner & Smith, 1992; Werner, 1993; Southwick & Charney, 2018) emphasize the role of people in the child's life who serve as what Alice Miller (1997) called "helping" or "enlightened" witnesses. These people (e.g., parents of friends, coaches, teachers, and others who actively step in) validate the child's experiences, support them, and mentor them. Such positive, involved role models and influencers, who treat an ACEIP with affection and respect in childhood, reassure them that they are intrinsically valuable and that help is available.

Internalizer children play a role in finding their helpers. Their sensitivity, perceptiveness, and desire to connect make them responsive to interest and potential support, helping set up a positive feedback loop that encourages the mentor's continued participation and interest. Even if their parents can't respond to them at a deep enough level, such children often find other nurturing and positive role models with whom to connect.

Understanding What Internalizing ACEIPs Need

When an internalizer ACEIP comes to you for therapy, their problems often center around a serious mismatch between their emotional needs and the self-absorption of the EI people in their life. Preparatory to learning how you can help internalizing ACEIPs, let's consider their most common motivations and personal needs.

Drive to Thrive

Most human beings seek ways to thrive, not just survive, and we all feel a boost from fulfilling our potential. Therefore, we are attracted to anything that lifts our spirits, raises our hopes, or gives us energy. Feeling good makes us feel more aware and alive. Every living thing reaches out toward opportunities for more growth.

EI parents are often quite controlling of, and even competitive with, their children, so they can have a hard time supporting each child's unique development. The EI parent wants their child to thrive, but only in the ways they approve of. Many ACEIPs end up feeling restricted, or like they haven't lived up to their potential.

Need to Love Others

Healthy humans have the capacity to love others in a multitude of forms. As we mature, our love can expand into an altruistic concern for others, especially our children. The well-being of the other person becomes a primary mission, and their survival can be as important as our own.

For ACEIPs, this capacity for loyalty beyond the self can paradoxically have harmful repercussions if they bond with EI people, groups, and ideas that emphasize self-sacrifice as the price of acceptance and connection. ACEIPs can idealistically over-identify with an EIP's outlook to the point that they lose sight of their own needs. Regarding EI parents, an ACEIP's *healing fantasies* keep hope alive that the parent will finally be able to connect emotionally and realize how important the relationship is.

Ultimately, ACEIPs face a reckoning when the costs of relationships with EIPs begin to exhaust their energy and hope. That can be the moment when people seek therapy—when they're feeling low, their minds are confused, and they're experiencing inner conflict between their needs and others' demands. Love and loyalty have depleted them, and the costs of self-sacrifice are mounting up.

Need to Feel Loved

Love goes beyond the primitive bonding that naturally takes place when people interact over time under conditions of familiarity and proximity (Bowlby, 1969/1982). Love means someone delights in your existence, feels joy in your presence, finds beauty in your being. Love tells you you're valued for who you are, making you feel special because your individuality is prized by another person. You become irreplaceable and crucial to their well-being, and they to yours. You become more of yourself through feeling accepted, knowing others, and being known. Unfortunately, this emotional recognition is something EIPs have trouble with, so the ACEIP "knows" they are loved, but they don't *feel* it.

An ACEIP who seeks therapy—your client—is someone who's been disappointed, hurt, or unseen in one of the most important and foundational relationships in their lives—their relationship with a parent. Perhaps they've gotten the idea that they're not enough or that they have disappointed the parent. Instead of feeling seen and known in this foundational relationship, ACEIPs have felt an odd blend of being emotionally overlooked, yet scrutinized for not quite measuring up. Without that early feeling of unconditional parental acceptance and emotional attunement, an ACEIP can be haunted all their life by vague fears of abandonment, unworthiness, or powerlessness (Firman & Gila, 1997).

Let me emphasize the critical psychological importance of *feeling seen*. From late infancy, we all sense our individuality. Later, this will develop into a defined sense of self and a conscious self-concept, but at the beginning of life, our nascent self needs to feel deeply good, lovable, and worthy of wholehearted attention from others. We need to know that our loved ones appreciate us in all our uniqueness, finding us interesting and adorable. I hope you can offer that appreciation for your clients' individuality. Believe me, they still need it, even after all these years. It's at the heart of ACEIP recovery.

When an immature parent's psychological limitations make it hard for them to emotionally welcome their child, this lack of response can shake the child's emerging self-image and self-confidence. A parent who holds back or criticizes instead of expressing love and acceptance creates a profound rift in their attunement with the child. With emotionally immature parents, children often grow up doubting whether their authentic self is acceptable. To not feel loved for who you are feels shaming. It's a judgment about your very worth. This is both shocking and humiliating to a child.

Feelings of humiliation are often followed by desperate efforts to make oneself into the kind of person that will hold the parent's favor. Instead of developing naturally within the safety of a relationship with a parent who knows and loves the child for themselves, the child works to construct a *false self* (Winnicott, 1989), designed to ingratiate them with the parent and protect them from further rejection and humiliation. They learn that constant vigilance and emotional work are the price of inclusion with other people.

Healing fantasies help an ACEIP take the sting out of these painful experiences, as they hold out hope that their EI parent will one day want to reach out for a deeper connection. But these fantasies don't help the ACEIP come to grips with the reality of their EIP's emotional limitations, to grieve their losses, and to find more responsive people.

Your awareness of these emotional injuries is important because your secretly humiliated, inadequately loved ACEIP client will need your utmost consideration as the background tone for their healing. Their innate dignity as a unique individual needs to be recognized and supported with warmth and respectful attention. As therapy progresses and you explore the roots of your client's self-doubt, they will become able to see what happened to them and stop judging themselves with such shame.

Need for Individuality and Connection

With confidence in our *individuality*, we can feel entitled to our own thoughts and feelings and can be clear about our psychological boundaries. And through deep *connection* with others, our individuality doesn't come at the cost of not belonging. We all need to maintain this balance between needing to belong and needing to be our unique selves. But EI parents often make their children feel that, in order to belong, they must suppress their autonomy and individuality. For them, connection has meant inhibiting themselves.

The child who grows up with an adequately emotionally mature parent doesn't feel forced to choose between belonging or being themselves. Similarly, the ACEIP client with a respectful, compassionate therapist will gradually learn that being oneself doesn't have to threaten one's connections. Such a therapist gives them the gift of a relationship with someone who encourages and supports their ability to know their own mind and be their true self.

Need for Empathy and Mirroring

Human connection involves receiving and giving *empathic* understanding. Not only does empathy feel reassuring and connecting, it directly helps a developing child learn about themselves through the emotional feedback of others.

We sense others' understanding in the way their facial expressions reflect our emotional experience. Our brains' *mirror neurons* (Rizzolatti, 2005; Rizzolatti & Craighero, 2004) subliminally take on others' facial and behavioral expressions and attune us to them at a deep, unconscious level. Synchronous feelings of connection register as the other person literally "mirrors" our posture or mood, making us feel accepted and understood. As a therapist, your awareness of mirroring makes you aware of the nonverbal signals you and your client are sending each other, showing you the quality of your mutual attunement in the moment. If an ACEIP client doesn't discern clear signals of empathy or mirroring from you, their default impression won't be that you are neutral—they will wonder what they're doing wrong.

After growing up with EI parents who didn't make them feel fully accepted, ACEIPs are unusually alert to any signs that another person is not in sync with them. Seeking reassurance becomes part of their communication style ("If that makes sense…"; "You know?"), just to make sure you're still listening to what they're saying. These verbalizations are also a way of equivocating on the authentic thing they just said, so it won't embarrass them if you don't get it. In therapy, this tentative, questioning tone may drop out once they get used to the unusual experience of truly being listened to by a kind, attentive person.

Need to Know Their Motives Are Understood

We all want to know that other people are interested and care enough to try to *mentalize* (Fonagy et al., 2002) our subjective experiences by imagining our unique inner perspective. Our ability to do so is based on our *theory of mind* (Premack & Woodruff, 1978; Baron-Cohen et al., 2000)—our realization that others possess a mind and viewpoints, just like we do. This awareness of others' mental activity starts early in humans. ACEIPs want to know not only that others feel for them, but also that their needs and motives are *understandable* to others; this reassures them they are not psychologically alone in this world.

Motivational understanding is a little different from empathy or mentalization; it's our ability to conceptualize what motivates people to feel, think, or act in certain ways. It deduces that others' needs and actions have purpose. When an EI parent is not aware of what motivates their child, they can't help their child to make sense of themselves. Children don't know why they have the urge to do something, or why they may go after something despite the consequences. Parents have to teach their children this deeper self-awareness by sharing their adult understanding. But since EI parents avoid emotional intimacy and meaningful conversations, they're not interested in helping their children consider their motives. Instead, they react to their children's behavior based on how it affected *them*. Without motivational understanding or interest, they make the child feel like there is something faulty in them for acting as they do, by saying things like: "Why did you do that?" "What's the matter with you?" or "Stop it!"

When a parent shows that they understand their child's motive, even if they can't condone the choice or behavior ("I know you were just trying to have fun, but…"), the child feels morally supported and no harm is done to their self-esteem. Parents who think about motives teach their children that their inner world makes sense and their actions have meaning. If a parent didn't do this for an ACEIP, you as therapist can. When you show motivational understanding of your clients, you are teaching them to be curious about why they do things. They learn from you how to understand their motives with interest and compassion.

Need for Existential Comfort and Meaning

Existential security is the feeling that the world makes sense and is hospitable to our existence. Our sense of life's meaning is based in feeling connected to others (Dowds, 2021). People can experience a deep loneliness and absence of meaning when not feeling known by and connected to others. And sometimes our capacity for abstract thinking can make this worse.

for her. Conventional talk therapy had not helped her much, so one day, I sat down with her and drew out a diagram of how I thought some of her traumatic experiences had sensitized her mind and preoccupied her attention. My client brightened immediately: now her intense sensitivity made sense to her, and she felt relief from the shaming idea that something was innately wrong with her. She kept that piece of paper in her purse and would pull it out whenever she started to get down on herself for her reactivity. Psychoeducation had given her more relief than anything else to that point.

I have found that when I explore the concept of emotional immaturity with ACEIP clients, it often clicks with them. Not only do my observations resonate with them, they also tend to open up more after gaining this insight. Positive feedback from readers of my books further confirms that people feel empowered by psychoeducation. However, although talking about emotional immaturity and EI parents can be an invaluable part of ACEIP therapy, it's best to offer it tentatively at first as a theory for the client to consider. Many ACEIP clients beginning therapy are quite protective of their parents and may not be immediately receptive to these ideas; it's important to be respectful and sensitive to how this information is landing with them.

Introducing the idea of emotional immaturity in loved ones is often more palatable to clients than labelling their loved one with a clinical diagnosis, such as one of the personality disorders. The rule of thumb is that all personality disorders are probably emotionally immature, but not all EI people qualify for a mental disorder diagnosis (American Psychiatric Association, 2013).

EIPs' Difficulty with Emotional Regulation and Stress Tolerance

Responsive parenting early in life gives us the baseline of empathy, security, and mutual respect that we need in all our deep relationships. Unfortunately, EI parents can actually feel threatened by their child's emotional needs. Instead of being able to calm and settle their child, EI parents themselves get upset by their child's emotions. An ACEIP's childhood needs for emotional intimacy and empathic parental responses often clash with their parent's defensive efforts to protect themselves from stress and emotional overload. This emotional mismatch between a child needing comfort and a poorly regulated, easily overwhelmed parent is a common issue for ACEIPs coming to see you in therapy.

Four Types of Emotionally Immature Parents

To better understand EI parent-child relationships and what they cost your client, let's review the four psychological styles of emotionally immature parents: emotional, rejecting, driven, and passive (Gibson, 2015). Each of these has a different maladaptive style of handling stress.

The **emotional type** of EI parent is volatile and shows intense emotions. They are highly reactive, with bursts of uncontrolled, unregulated affect. They're so insecure that they exaggerate threats and suspect betrayals in their relationships, overreacting to the tiniest hint of rejection. They desperately crave love but are so intense that other people want to get away from them. When threatened or held to account, they reflexively project blame onto others. Using guilt and shame, they make others feel responsible for their unhappiness. Everything is somebody else's fault.

Their children grew up walking on eggshells around a scary adult whose emotions ruled all and who acted vulnerable and victimized. With this kind of parent, your client's childhood was overshadowed by parental emotional instability, impulsivity, outbursts, or acting out, often against a backdrop of chronic depression or anxiety. The emotional type of parent can't see past their own upset to consider how their children feel or are affected by their lack of emotional control.

The **rejecting type** of parent looms over a family like a menacing thundercloud. They avoid closeness with their children and make them feel like a burden, as if they're always bothering or displeasing the parent. Such parents stay to themselves, radiating the threat of anger if disturbed. They usually keep their feelings under wraps and aren't invested in complaining to others—they're not inhibited; they just don't see the point of sharing. This ominous parent wants to be served while being spared the expectation of any emotional reciprocity. Even if they never turn abusive, there is always a mood of volcanic anger, spite, or hatred waiting to erupt. The rejecting type isn't interested in parenting and was rarely invested in being a parent in the first place.

The **driven type** of EI parent is likely to be seen as exemplary. They're intelligent, motivated, socially adapted people who stay busy and goal-directed at all times. They seem perfectly adjusted and very invested in their children's activities and success. They are always accomplishing something and find security in excelling or being thought well of. It's nearly impossible for them to slow down long enough to really listen to their child or be present for their deep feelings. Emotional intimacy is rare with the time-conscious driven parent. The driven type can't emotionally nurture because their own agendas keep them too busy to tune in to what their children may be experiencing.

With this parent, your ACEIP client may feel an odd blend of knowing that they were well cared for physically and socially, while being emotionally lonely. Since social status and occupational prestige rank so highly with these driven parents, your client may pressure and overextend themselves, as though constantly trying to measure up.

The **passive type** of EI parent seems more benign and is often the parent to whom your client felt closest. Passive types aren't as unstable, judgmental, or pressured as the other types, and the friendlier ones seem warm and pleasant to be around. They often pair with one of the more dominant EI types to start their family, so by comparison, they seem like the kinder, emotionally safer parent.

Even though passive types can be more responsive and even playful, they are still emotionally immature, showing basic egocentrism, limited empathy, and an unwillingness to protect their child from the damaging effects of the other parent. The passive parent sidesteps parental responsibilities by allowing the other parent to rule the roost. Though pleasant, they avoid emotional intimacy or genuine interest in others, tuning out inconvenient or upsetting realities. While they may be comforting at times, it is usually at low cost to them and doesn't involve real listening or protectiveness. Passive types are more like big kids or adolescents who just don't feel accountable for the safety or emotional health of their children. They focus on what they want to do and assume everything else will take care of itself.

Your client's parents might have shown combinations or varying degrees of these characteristics. But an EI parent will usually fall mostly under one category because each type shows unique psychological defenses and coping.

Marriages can bring together different types, but as family therapist Murray Bowen (1978) noted, people of similar levels of emotional maturity and psychological individuation tend to end up with each other regardless of personality type. (Marriages tend not to last between an EI person and a partner who is developing emotional maturity. Their sensitivities and world views would become too different.)

If you, as therapist, realize how depriving this lack of parental emotional sensitivity feels, you'll be able to use your empathic understanding to help your ACEIP clients find themselves again. In the rest of this chapter, we'll look at how the defensiveness and rigid brain style of an EI parent can rebuff the emotional and existential needs of your ACEIP client—and how you can help them with that. Jackie's story, below, shows what it's like for an ACEIP as they struggle to understand a parent's emotional immaturity.

Jackie's Story

Jackie was the responsible eldest daughter of an emotionally immature mother. She had never understood why her mother couldn't see how destructive and self-centered her behavior often was. As the oldest, Jackie felt responsible for everyone, but her siblings—who didn't feel a similar caretaker responsibility— took a lighter approach, brushing off the absurdity of their mother's attitudes at times with, "Oh, you know how Mom is!" Jackie wished she could let her mother's behavior roll off her back too, but she couldn't shake the belief that her mother could change if she wanted to.

Jackie was interested in growth and self-awareness, and she was sure her mother must have some potential for that. It was hard for her to think of her mother's limitations in terms of emotional immaturity. She'd think, *I want to see if this time, she might get it.* Jackie firmly believed that people could be communicated with and change. Accepting her mother's limitations felt like a dereliction of duty. "What's the difference between 'accepting' and 'giving up'?" Jackie wondered aloud to me. "I don't want to give up on my mother and be left feeling like I didn't try hard enough."

When Jackie was growing up, she wanted to help make things better in the family. She took her responsibility deeply to heart but was repeatedly dismayed by her mother's self-centered behavior. Jackie kept trying to reach her mother, but her mother showed no desire to talk about anything at a deeper level. Instead of having real conversations with Jackie, her mother focused on "fluff and talking about other people." In Jackie's words, "She won't do any emotional work; I'm doing it for both of us. She's not thinking about me, and if she is, it's something like, 'Oh, I wonder what she's having for dinner tonight.'"

As long as Jackie was using herself as her basis to try to understand her mother, she was going to be frustrated and confused. Things became clearer to her when she learned about emotional immaturity and the fundamental differences it creates between people. Let's dive in for a deeper look at the causes and manifestations of this immaturity.

We all recognize childish behavior in adults. Not only have we *seen* it before, we've all *done* it before. When we're not at our best or we're feeling strained, we can lapse into EI behaviors. However, there are seven hallmark characteristics of EIPs that define more entrenched emotional immaturity. I'll describe them below; you can print out checklists for your clients to complete at http://www.newharbinger.com/53592.

Seven Hallmark Characteristics of EIPs

1. EIPs are egocentric
2. EIPs have limited empathy
3. EIPs are not self-reflective
4. EIPs fear emotional intimacy
5. EIPs deny, dismiss, and distort reality, on the basis of their feelings
6. EIPs have a one-sided view of relationships
7. EIPs show mental rigidity

1. EIPs Are Egocentric

EIPs are, first and foremost, extremely self-preoccupied and exhibit the kind of all-encompassing egocentricity that is usually found in children. Think about the typical three- or four-year-old and how completely focused they are on their own needs and pleasures. They just don't have the maturity to consider other people's inner experiences or rights. Both EIPs and preschoolers believe that their urgent needs should come first.

It's normal for toddlers to be egocentric because they're trying to establish their own identity. They have to be self-centered because they're in the process of developing their individuality. But EIPs get stuck at this developmental task, and instead of evolving a secure inner sense of self to give them security and identity, they regulate their emotions and fragile self-image by following their emotions and impulses. Like young children, EIPs have not yet fully developed their sense of self.

We usually think of narcissism or grandiosity when we consider egocentrism, but a person can also be extremely self-centered around their issues of anxiety, insecurity, or low self-esteem. Whether domineering or dependent, an EI parent can't be there for their child's emotional needs. The style of an EIP's egocentrism may vary, but it still communicates the message that nobody else's needs are as important. Neither type experiences other people's inner worlds as psychologically real (Anderson, 1995; Shaw, 2014) and they pursue their agendas regardless of the effect on others. For example:

- A mother who changes the subject from her child's problem to her own concerns

- A father who threatens disinheritance when his son refuses to join the family business

- A depressed parent who makes cynical comments when their child is enthusiastic

2. EIPs Have Limited Empathy

An EIP's self-centeredness means they have poor empathy, neither imagining nor feeling another person's subjective experience. If they're feeling satisfied and well-resourced at the moment, EIPs may show some fleeting empathy. But it's not their natural orientation. Usually, they aren't interested in other people's points of view—unless they agree with them—and they find others' feelings irrelevant. Other people's inner experience just isn't real to an EIP.

This lack of empathy explains why EIPs often wade into conversations without concern for trampling on other people's values or viewpoints. They just assume everyone is—and should be—like them, despite any evidence to the contrary. They're not necessarily intending to start a fight when they say offensive things—although that's okay with them too. They just assume egocentrically that others are just like them and feel the same way they do. Their urge to express themselves trumps any discretion or consideration for others. Toddlers don't hold themselves back from immediate self-expression, and EIPs don't either. For the EIP and the young child, it begins and ends with: *Here's what I feel like saying now.* For example:

- An EI boss publicly yells at an employee for making a mistake.

- A mother tells a child's embarrassing story to others in front of them.

- A father doesn't notice what others see as his daughter's depressed behavior.

3. EIPs Are Not Self-Reflective

In optimal development, our brains constantly integrate our experiences into emotional memories that form our sense of self (Winnicott, 1989; Schore, 2012). Without this intrapsychic integration and empathy, EIPs lack the sense of self and observational stance enabling reflections on themselves and others. They can't step back and think about their own thinking in that kind of "meta" way that would allow them to be both the observer and the person observed.

Without the ability to meta-process our own experiences, there is no curiosity about one's self or motives, and usually no motivation for change. Deeper reflection doesn't occur to such a person: they are who they are, and that's that. So:

- They'll blame other people for everything and never wonder if they themselves are part of the problem.

- They believe bad things keep happening to them through no fault of their own.

- They don't stand back and reevaluate their parenting behavior.

4. EIPs Fear Emotional Intimacy

Emotional intimacy is created when people share their deep thoughts and feelings with each other. Emotional intimacy requires trusting the other person to "get" us. It deepens our relationships and makes us feel known by another person. Since these close moments can't be controlled or forced, such connections are even more meaningful when they happen.

However, EI people find emotional intimacy destabilizing; it's too deep and fluid to feel comfortable in. They prefer cut-and-dried rules, structure, and control to feel secure. To keep life securely simple, they may see their relationship with their child solely through family roles, rather than as two real people with subjective viewpoints and ever-changing inner worlds. In their family role, the child is reduced to playing a part in the EIP's life, with no acknowledgement of their own individual existence or motivations.

The child of such a parent finds that when they try to open up to their parent and share their inner experiences, their parent pulls back rather than engaging. A healthy parental response might show curiosity, acceptance, or interest, which would foster further communication. But EI parents tense up when things get real, even around impromptu expressions of love, finding them emotionally destabilizing. The child is left with the feeling that their openness went too far or even repulsed the parent. For example:

- A parent quickly changes the subject or scoffs when their child shows affection.

- The parent retreats emotionally or goes off on a tangent when their child tries to have an honest conversation with them.

- A mother makes fun of her son when he confesses his fears and tells him to "man up."

5. EIPs Deny, Dismiss, and Distort Reality Based on Their Feelings

EIPs often decipher reality on the basis of their feelings alone, insisting that reality is what they *feel* it is, regardless of facts. This is called *affective realism* (Barrett & Bar, 2009), a highly reactive, self-referential, and nonobjective approach to reality. With such emotionally based reality perception, EIPs' view of life reveals more about their unresolved emotional issues than what's really happening.

For instance, the EI parent might take a message like "Mom, when you don't listen to me, I feel frustrated," and pare it down to something that *feels* more true to them, like "So you're saying I don't love you?!" They think they are exposing a deeper truth when really all they are doing is jumping to conclusions, going to extremes, and changing the topic—in this case, pretending the issue is about love rather than communication.

Your ACEIP client also probably has had the experience of their parent's *dismissing* ("That's ridiculous! How silly!"), *denying* ("I never said that; that's crazy"), or *distorting* their perceptions ("You're remembering this all wrong; that's not how it happened, and even if it had, I would never have done that").

Gaslighting, the complete invalidation of someone's view of reality (Marlow-MaCoy, 2020), is easy for EIPs to use when things aren't going their way. Due to their parent's poor empathy and reality distortions, your ACEIP client may be especially vulnerable to gaslighting. They've been raised to second-guess and self-doubt their most basic experiences and feelings in such situations.

People can't have emotional intimacy or emotional closeness when they can't even agree on what happened between them, nor work out differences if the basic facts of a situation aren't mutually accepted. For example:

- A mother accuses her adult daughter of hating her when the daughter sets a boundary on the length of the mother's visits.

- A father flat-out denies he ever said something when you know you heard it.

- An EI boss forms the belief that someone is trying to make him look bad when it's not so.

6. EIPs Have a One-Sided View of Relationships

EIPs conduct themselves as the most important person in any relationship. They structure their relationships according to what I call an *emotionally immature relationship system* (EIRS). Any of their relationships that advance beyond social superficiality will show this pattern. For EIPs, the other person in their relationships is implicitly tasked with:

- Helping maintain the EIP's emotional stability

- Shoring up the EIP's vulnerable self-esteem

Other people are expected to soothe them when they're upset, agree with them when they're angry, and calm them when they're anxious. Others also should be exquisitely attuned to their self-esteem, buffering them so they always feel competent and good about themselves. EIPs' relational attitudes are reminiscent of toddlers': *Always make me feel better; mirror my feelings and wishes; meet my needs; let me control you.* For example:

- A parent acts morally affronted when their adult child has a differing opinion.

- A partner expects their spouse to always build them up and never offer criticism or suggestions.

- A parent believes their adult child has a moral obligation to protect the parent's feelings no matter what.

7. EIPs Show Mental Rigidity

EIPs show inflexibility and a one-track mind instead of considering different viewpoints. They conceptualize life in extremes of black and white, good and bad. As a result, they are judgmental and claim unjustified certainty in their opinions. Also, due to their poorly integrated sense of self, they can hold mutually contradictory ideas, not having enough internal consistency to notice they're not making sense.

With little concern over plausibility or reasonableness, they unthinkingly say and do things that don't fit together, and are not troubled by cognitive dissonance (Festinger, 1957/1985). This results in what looks like hypocritical or illogical behavior to other people. So:

- Even when an EIP's assertions are disproved, they might insist, "I know what I saw."

- An EIP will insist right is right and wrong is wrong, even if there are clearly mitigating circumstances.

- Social roles are sacrosanct to an EIP; people are respected for their status, not their behavior.

Next, we'll go into more detail about how the EIP's brain style contributes to their generally defensive orientation toward life.

EIPs' Left-Brain-Hemisphere Traits

Ideally, the two hemispheres of our brains work together seamlessly in an integrated way, giving us the advantage of two minds in one. Optimal cognitive and emotional functioning depends on this integrated brain function. Internalizer ACEIPs are much more likely than EIPs to have integrated minds, with both right- and left-brain capacities. Therapy aims to develop this brain balance further.

However, many cognitive characteristics of EIPs are similar to traits of people who show more dominant left-brain-hemisphere functioning (McGilchrist, 2009, 2021; Tweedy, 2021). Brain laterality is enormously complex and unfortunately has often been oversimplified into stereotypical and thus inaccurate depictions of personality. However, research on hemispheric brain damage or temporary suppression of brain-hemisphere function (see McGilchrist, 2021, for a comprehensive review) does show there are significant functional hemispheric differences. Some of the most salient differences lie in the *ways* people perceive and attend to reality. We need both hemispheres working together; aside from specialized tasks, people tend to function less well in the world when they rigidly over-emphasize one hemisphere over the other.

The left-brain hemisphere is clever and reductive. It analyzes, breaks things down into parts, and sees the world as a mechanical system that operates sequentially. In contrast, the right-brain hemisphere is comprehensive and integrative. It looks for complex connections within the big picture, and is attuned to empathy and respect between people and the living world.

As psychiatrist and scholar Iain McGilchrist (2009, 2021) points out, left-brain-hemisphere dominance means that a person's worldview is sliced and diced into details, categories, and rigid belief systems. Even when the evidence is right before them, a left hemisphere-dominant person (like many EIPs) summarily rejects reality if it clashes with their preconceived beliefs. This narrowmindedness and oversimplification contribute to the reality distortions of EIPs, promoting anger and irritability when crossed.

Personality Correlates of Left-Hemisphere Dominance

Jumping to conclusions and thinking that you know everything is associated with a left brain–dominant view of the world. Such an outlook sees others' viewpoints as irrelevant. Without the benefit of right-brained global insights and integrative thinking, they overlook complex patterns of influence and meaningful connections.

As brain researchers have noted, the left-hemisphere viewpoint doesn't know what it doesn't know—due to its tunnel vision—but it's sure its opinion is the whole story. For the left brain–dominant person, reality is what *they* say it is. You can't be curious about or receptive to others' thoughts if you already know all there is to know. EIPs' rigidity and egocentric confidence prompt them to give advice and push ideas even when they know less than other people.

Understanding left-brained attitudes might help your internalizer ACEIP client take it less personally when the EIPs in their life dismiss them, distort their intent, or don't listen to them.

Perhaps many EIPs stay in their left brains so much to give themselves a sense of control and certainty. Unfortunately, this cuts them off from the benefits of right-brained feelings of empathy and shared experiences, losing the opportunity for the little connections with others that offer emotional nurturance. It's as if their social engagement systems are frequently offline. When their child scans their face for a sense of reciprocity and connection, the EI parent is often too tense or too self-preoccupied to respond with emotional connection cues, which causes uneasiness and even distress in their child (see *still-face experiments* in Tronick, 2007); for videos, search YouTube for "Tronick still-face experiments" and "The Problem of Disconnection: The Still Face Experiment" (Puder, 2019).

EIPs' Feelings of Unsafety and Defensiveness

The compulsively defensive and rigidly self-protective attitudes of EIPs hint at chronic insecurity and feelings of unsafety. Two concepts, polyvagal theory and transgenerational pain, help explain why their defensive reactions are so strong.

EIP Defensiveness and the Polyvagal Theory

While the *sympathetic nervous system* prepares us for fight or flight, the *parasympathetic system* slows us down. Each of these systems in the autonomic nervous system can either initiate constructive action or react intensely to threat. Whether EIPs respond through their sympathetic or parasympathetic systems, they react instantly to feeling threatened.

The long, branching vagus nerve extends throughout the body and is a main component of the parasympathetic nervous system. This vagal nerve governs some very different functions, such as: rest and relaxation, facilitating social engagement and support with others, and, in the face of extreme shock or threat to life, immobilization. Neuroscientist Stephen Porges's (2011) *polyvagal theory* has theorized that two different pathways within the vagus nerve are responsible for these very different parasympathetic tasks and states of being.

The *ventral* pathway of the vagus nerve activates feelings of safety, calm, relaxation, and connection to others: what Porges calls our *social engagement system.* It helps us notice and respond to social and affectional cues, such as a welcoming and reassuring tone of voice, eye contact, reassuring touch, and face-to-face mirroring—all of which are sources of connection and, hence, safety.

The *dorsal* vagal pathway is very different; it takes over when we're under extreme threat, triggering a shutdown response. This causes us to "freeze" or dissociate, which is our primal, last-ditch reaction to imminent threat. The perceived dangers that trigger this shutdown can be psychological, just as much as physical.

Often, when EIPs should be open to emotional engagement, they react to closeness as if under threat. They either withdraw and freeze up (parasympathetic), or become defensive, evasive, and critical (sympathetic). Their emotional anxieties make it hard for them to feel safe in these moments of connection; they can't relax their guard long enough to enjoy relaxed and open relationships with others. Instead, they try to keep it superficial or assert control.

Perhaps due to earlier trauma or other experiences, EIPs' capacity for deep connection with others seems stunted and fraught with anxiety. They act as though emotional connection would leave them defenseless against let-down, abandonment, or outright attack. Consequently, openness and emotional intimacy—even with their own children—feels unsafe. They dissociate or shut down just when their children need them the most. When the child needs supportive ventral vagal engagement from their EI parent, they can get dorsal vagal shutdown instead.

EIP Defensiveness and Transgenerational Pain

We can't know all of what EIPs went through in their early lives that could've shut down their emotional engagement with others. Perhaps they had attachment disruptions (Ainsworth et al., 1974; Ainsworth, 1982; Wallin, 2007/2015) or experienced trauma, abuse, or deprivation. Whether the causes were nature- or nurture-based, or a mixture, EI parents seem to pass down their own difficult emotional experiences to their children (Wolynn, 2016), perpetuating a transgenerational inheritance of emotional reactivity and emotional loneliness.

With possible traumas and deprivation in their past, EIPs' capacity for emotional self-regulation is easily overwhelmed, coming out in unmodulated and volatile ways. Their emotional expression tends more toward fear and anger than love, trust, or connection. This reflected pain can get passed down the generations through children modeling their parent's (often subconscious) reactions (Bandura, 1971/2017).

Understanding Helps with Acceptance

Jackie, whom we met earlier, was able to integrate her understanding of emotional immaturity into her relationship with her mother. Here's what that looked like.

Accepting Emotional Immaturity Characteristics As Jackie talked about her frustration with her mother, we identified how her mother showed emotionally immature characteristics. This gave Jackie some intellectual distance from the high reactivity she often had toward her mother's exasperating behavior.

Accepting Differences in Reality Orientation While Jackie intellectually agreed that her mother fit these characteristics of emotional immaturity, there was a hitch. "What right do I have to say that my reality is more real than hers?" Jackie wondered, trying to be fair to her mother. "That's a good question," I said. "Can you answer it?" Jackie thought a moment and said, "Maybe my reality *is* accurate. But it's not a good feeling to feel smarter than your parent. I don't want to be more mature than my mom."

At that moment, Jackie was speaking from her inner-child part who hated to think that her mother was not the wise adult who always knew best. But as soon as Jackie heard herself speaking this childhood fear out loud, she backtracked and admitted, "I really *do* know reality better and in a fuller way than my mom." Jackie now realized how tired she was of deferring to her mother's emotional distortions so as not to threaten her young self's need to have a mother with greater maturity. Jackie's began to give up this old hope once she stated it aloud and could hear how untrue it was. (We'll see more about how that works in chapter 10.)

Jackie was beginning to come to grips with her mother's emotional immaturity in a realistic and helpful way: "I wish that wasn't my life story. I wish I could have fulfilling discussions with my mother like I have with my kids. But she has no idea there's a deeper reality than surface things. She still surprises me: I just can't believe she can't do it." As Jackie increased her knowledge of emotional immaturity, she could gradually release her wishful fantasies about her mom's capacity for change.

Accepting Cognitive Differences As Jackie and I worked through her emotional resistance to seeing her mom's mental and emotional limitations, we also discussed possible differences in their brain function. Jackie seemed to have much more right- and left-brain integration than her mother, giving Jackie insight and self-reflection. Her mother was apparently missing those skills.

One day I asked Jackie how it would affect her view of her mother if she found out that all this time her mother had had a cognitive limitation that made it impossible for her to feel and think more deeply. What if she saw her mother as an unimaginative person with limited interests who simply didn't have the complexity to hear what Jackie was trying to tell her? Metaphorically, what if Jackie was a naturally three-dimensional person, and her mother was naturally two-dimensional? Just considering this idea gave Jackie some much-needed relief from trying so hard to get her mother to understand. Her lingering childhood view of her mother as all-powerful and omniscient was beginning to adjust to realities that Jackie now could begin to accept.

Understanding Brain Styles, Emotional Needs, and Individuality

Understanding the differences between left brain–dominant and more integrated minds can give ACEIPs perspective on their EI parent's deficits as caregivers. Since EIPs often favor left-brained rigidity and judgment, EI parents are especially likely to make ACEIPs feel bad about a) their emotional needs and b) their desire to assert their individuality.

The right brain supports empathy, emotional resonance, and appreciation of individuality (McGilchrist, 2021). Knowing their EI parent is poorly equipped for these functions can give ACEIPs insight into why they don't feel understood or seen by the parent at an emotional level. Realizing that a parent might have trouble accessing the part of their minds needed for close relationships and processing emotions—that their indifference or refusal to listen may be partly *cognitive*—helps your client realize that perhaps the parent just wasn't able to reciprocate. Confirming the healthiness and wholeness of their own emotional process helps restore ACEIPs' self-esteem and self-confidence.

The Beauty of Our Right Hemisphere

The right hemisphere of our brain is attuned to subtle and tender emotions (McGilchrist, 2021). Resonance between parent and child's limbic centers and right hemisphere brain forms the child's original primal bonds (Lewis et al., 2000; Schore, 2009, 2022). Through mutual activation of their right hemispheres and emotional centers, parent and child synchronize their facial expressions and body cues, letting each other know that they're attuned to them (Tronick, 2007). This provides the relational predictability and sense of oneness that babies need as the foundation of their security in the world.

Much research has shown the right hemisphere isn't just a warm and fuzzy nicety; it supplies us with an intuitive, integrative, and wholistic perspective on reality (McGilchrist, 2021). With it, we *experience* another person's presence and realness, while the left hemisphere tends to flatten and narrow our view of others, perceiving them as objects or functions. The right hemisphere sees things in context, senses relationships and connections, registers overall context, and grasps meaningful gestalts instead of disassembled parts. Originality, human relationships, artistic expression, and invention are its natural strong suits. When we learn something, our right hemisphere integrates new and old information into higher levels of comprehension. With its sensitivity to emotion and capacity for insight, you might say the right brain is made for psychotherapy.

Unlike the left, the right hemisphere doesn't need to be right all the time. It keeps seeking truth (Taylor, J. B., 2021) and readily adapts if a better idea emerges. It is attracted to complexity, and grasps the tone, implications, and mood of other people's communications. This receptivity and curiosity promote emotional maturation and deep relationships.

Based on its emotionally informed experience, the right hemisphere uses symbols and imagery to grasp things instantly and empathically, while the left brain's style is more explicit, verbal, logical, and sequential. The right brain finds connections that spark creativity and lightbulb moments; the left hemisphere marches stepwise through grids of explicit, concrete data. If the left brain is definitive and exclusive (either/or), the right hemisphere finds similarities, connections, meanings, and relationships (both/and). We wouldn't be able to function well without them both, but while the right brain understands the talents of the left, the left often disdains what the right has to offer.

Offering Attunement and Right-Brain Understanding

If your ACEIP client has grown up with an EI parent who had an unempathic left-brain orientation, imagine what it will mean to that client when you listen with your right-brain emotional awareness and openness to whatever they want to tell you. For an ACEIP, the therapy invitation to talk about whatever's important to them is a profoundly validating experience. They can just be themselves and let their feelings lead the way. This is a

livelihood or accomplishments. As situations require, such a person can relate to others flexibly in appropriately dependent, independent, or interdependent ways. Their capacity for love includes the crucial capacity to see other people as psychologically real (Anderson, 1995) and as individuals in their own right, thereby making possible respect, empathy, and real emotional intimacy. They make other people feel seen, safe, and comfortable being themselves. Their ability to work means they can achieve adequate self-sufficiency, and they have the ability to take on adult responsibilities in society. So:

- They are able to see others as psychologically real and worthy of respect.

- They show both self-reliance and emotional bonding with others.

- They can pursue their own goals and consider the needs of others at the same time.

Ability to Self-Regulate and Tolerate Stress Sufficiently emotionally mature people can manage their emotional reactions to stress, consider which responses would be most adaptive, and use both thinking and feeling skills to meet life's challenges. Stress is hard on everyone, but adequately emotionally mature people don't become psychologically disorganized, emotionally dysregulated, or unfairly blame others when things get tense. They feel things deeply in a complex way, but usually aren't incapacitated by the intensity of their emotions. They might feel temporarily overwhelmed, but they bounce back. They use mature coping mechanisms that assess and adapt to reality rather than struggling against it (Vaillant, G. E., 2000). For example:

- Stress prompts them to slow down and think things out, rather than react impulsively.

- They seek input from others when unsure of themselves, and listen carefully so they can widen their consideration of all factors.

- Instead of insisting that reality should change to make them more comfortable, they seek advantageous ways to adapt to changed realities.

Chapter Wrap-Up

Understanding EIPs' characteristics through psychoeducation mitigates their impact on your ACEIP client. EIPs' main traits include: emotional dysregulation, low stress tolerance, immature coping mechanisms, egocentrism, low empathy, poor self-reflection, reality distortions, one-sided relationships, and mental rigidity—which may reflect a lack of brain hemisphere integration. The four types of EI parents—emotional, rejecting, driven, and passive—are not able to give their children adequate empathy or deep enough emotional connection for secure and healthy relationships. There are probably multiple possible roots of emotional immaturity, but traits of emotional maturity are generally the same across people. As ACEIP clients learn to identify these trait qualities of their EIPs, especially in contrast to emotional maturity, they lessen their reactivity to these behaviors. To help our clients at a deep enough level, we need techniques that work with not only explicit memories, but deep implicit learnings as well. Adequately emotionally mature people show adaptability by processing complex circumstances and emotional stress while still being able to love and work.

Keep in Mind

- ACEIPs can take things less personally if they understand the EIP's developmental limitations.

- Left brain–dominant EIPs keep emotional distance by focusing on supposed "facts" and ignoring emotional content.

- When recalling and verbalizing explicit memories don't seem to help the client's problem, look for implicit emotional memories governing their interpersonal patterns.

- There's no downside to validating a client's inner world. It may seem distorted or need to be healed, but it's generally a map to their early emotional experiences.

Chapter 3

The Psychological Cost of Relationships with EIPs

EIPs typically haven't developed internally enough to have a secure inner sense of self, so they depend on others—including their children—to stabilize their emotions and self-esteem. In relationships, EIPs are like young children who need others to mirror them and reinforce their security and sense of goodness. Consequently, family members are valued for what they can provide to EIPs' security and self-pride, not for their own individuality.

EIPs experience their children as extensions of themselves. Respectful personal boundaries therefore don't make sense to them. They feel entitled to direct their child in all ways, frequently invalidating the child's sense of self and experience of reality. Instead of helping their child form their own personality, the EI parent often emotionally enmeshes with their child and expects the child to mirror and validate the parent's egocentric view of the world. It just wouldn't occur to an EI parent to wonder how their child feels about things.

To them, children exist as family roles and are seen as part of the "undifferentiated family ego mass" (Bowen, 1978), which is a conglomeration of parents' projections and expectations. This pressure for *enmeshment* and identity-sharing constricts your ACEIP client's sense of self and entitlement to their own individuality. Treated as more of a possession or filling a familial role than an emerging individual, it's been existentially hard for your ACEIP client to see themselves as entitled to their own feelings, thoughts, and individuality.

The Coercive Ploys of EIPs

EIPs' self-centeredness drives their need to be the center of everyone's attention and concern. They have learned that using coercive ploys often makes other people back off or give them what they want.

Emotional Takeovers and Distortion Fields

An *emotional takeover* is when an EIP's emotional demands override other people's priorities and preferences. We could call this "manipulative," but that connotes too much consciousness. I think of it more as the reflexive reaction of an immature psychological system facing a stress it can't manage. Once you placate and indulge the upset EIP, they begin to calm down, just like little kids do.

EIPs also stir up what psychologist Brian Wald has called *distortion fields*: episodes of urgent emotional upheaval in which they insist that other people treat their emotional distress as an emergency requiring immediate attention. For instance, they might call in the middle of the night because they are drunk, lonely, having a panic attack, or got bad news that day—showing no awareness of your need for a full night's sleep.

One of the most helpful things you can do for your ACEIP client is to help them disengage from the tractor-beam of the EIP's emotional intensity. Help your client consider: *Is* it an emergency? *Does* it have to be solved right at that moment? *Do* you have to be the answer to their problem every time? Your client will feel pressured by the EIP, sure, but you can help them build new habits of objectivity and self-protection, such as setting limits on when they can be contacted or how long they will listen. Remind your client that the 911 dispatcher starts by saying, "911. What is your emergency?" because there'd better be a real emergency. Help your client learn to spot and refuse to be taken over by these boundary incursions.

Emotional Coercion

Another type of EI behavior that makes it hard for your ACEIP client to set limits with EIPs is *emotional coercion* (Gibson, 2019). These behaviors stir up guilt, shame, fear, or self-doubt in people, which makes ACEIPs doubt themselves and capitulate. Coercive EIPs instinctively know how to make others feel afraid, uncertain, or bad about themselves. Any assertive, self-protective, or independent moves by an ACEIP often will be branded as disloyalty or betrayal by the EIP. (From the EI perspective, anyone who thwarts their desires is by definition morally bad.)

———————Tyrone's Story———————

Fear is especially effective for coercion. For example, my client Tyrone had begun to resist his father's opinions and demands. But whenever Tyrone wanted to make his own decisions, his father threatened to withdraw his financial backing. His father frequently reminded him that he *did* have a right to comment on Tyrone's relationship and work choices because he paid for Tyrone's college and co-signed a loan for his first home, shaming Tyrone into feeling guilty for wanting autonomy. His father's threats scared Tyrone into tunnel vision—it felt to him as if his father's support was his only route to security and success.

Tyrone had learned to minimize his own needs and feelings to get along with his dad. Each time this came up, we focused in depth on how it felt to do that. By not discounting his feelings or glossing over his father's threats, Tyrone began to recognize how it felt to be treated that way. He became less willing to feel judged and coerced by his father. Ultimately, Tyrone was able to set calm limits with his father, ride out his threats, and make alternate plans, if necessary, for how to pursue his goals without his father's support. It was a small price to pay for no longer being his father's emotional hostage.

Emotional Attack

An *emotional attack* is when the EIP escalates from insidious pressure to outright bullying. For instance, an EIP decides the ACEIP did something wrong and deserves harsh words for being that way. Their tone is personal, more "You are stupid and wrong and need to change" than "I don't like what you did." Emotional attacks are aggressive, authoritarian, blunt, and unkind—pure criticism under a banner of superiority. The EI parent's externalization of blame and mistrust of others, including their children, teaches the child to mistrust their own perception if it differs from their parent's. The ACEIP thus loses faith in their own judgment.

Reactivity Fuels Emotional Enmeshment

Since many EI parents see other family members as extensions of themselves rather than as individuals with their own personalities, they don't see the need for personal boundaries (Tawwab, 2021). Such parents expect even their grown children to think the same way they do, and to have the same values and interests. This is often framed as "love" and "closeness," but EIPs are actually demanding that everyone be like them. Such enmeshment means that the EIP's needs should be everyone's problem, and that others are responsible for the EIP's feelings. If anyone tries to individuate (Bowen, 1978) from this family dynamic, other family members will often try to pressure the offender back in line just to keep the peace with the EIP.

EIPs use other people's *emotional reactivity* to gain control over situations. By provoking conflict or anger, they get the upper hand. EIPs expect other people to mirror them, to feel the same way they do and to believe the same things. If the other person won't do this voluntarily, the EIP will escalate in ways that pull the person into their emotional orbit involuntarily.

James's Story

James's father thought James should be more attentive to his mother. James had a difficult relationship with her and at times would have to take a break from their contact for a while. But if James didn't send a card or call his mom on a special day, his father would text him to remind and reprimand him. James, angry, felt pressured by his father to have a certain kind of relationship with his mother, whether he wanted to or not, and after a scolding, his father and mother occupied his thoughts for days. By trying to establish boundaries, he unfortunately felt more—not less—emotionally entangled with his parents.

But once James remained calm—noticing his parents' pressure but claiming freedom to make up his own mind—he exited the triangulated family dynamic of being the bad guy while his father played rescuer to his mother's hurt feelings (Karpman, 1968). James became able to tell his father that his relationship with his mother was not something he could discuss with him. James's calm resolve and neutral observation of his father's attempts to control him enabled him to keep his boundaries straight and not let his father dictate his actions.

EI parents maintain control and influence only as long as the ACEIP remains emotionally reactive to them. That's why it's crucial for your client to understand that EIPs' criticisms and outbursts serve a very specific purpose: to provoke the emotional reactivity that binds your client to them. Initially, Jackie, Tyrone, and James all couldn't resist reacting to their EI parents' behavior, but once they became aware of how reactivity undermined their autonomy, they found it easier to resist being drawn into emotional enmeshments they didn't want. They learned to stay in touch with themselves instead of getting reactive to the EIP's attempted coercions.

Once they're in the grip of an EIP's pressures and projections, it can be nearly impossible for ACEIPs to see what they're caught up in. Psychoeducation and an improved understanding of psychological dynamics can pull your client back from the brink of overinvolvement. Going into interactions with more self-awareness and objectivity (Gibson, 2015) helps them keep their footing.

Using Self-Awareness to Lower Emotional Reactivity

As a therapist, you can help your ACEIP client catch emotional reactivity early and use it as a signal to:

- back up and reconnect with their own thoughts and feelings

- practice dispassionate objectivity toward the EIP's emotional pressure

By practicing these two responses, your client can hold on to themselves amidst the EIP's smokescreen of emotionality and crisis, and remain objective in spite of the EIP's efforts to suck them into their perceived emergency. Teach your client to remain connected to their true self and grounded in their body by focusing on:

- slow, calming breaths

- mindful attentiveness to details of their surroundings

- feeling grounded and embodied

- stroking or stretching their arms or neck

- the sensation of their feet anchored to the floor

- surreptitiously contracting individual muscles in a deliberate way

- narrating their experiences to themselves

- taking breaks away from the tense situation for a few moments

Reactivity always feels compulsive—like you have no choice but to feel a certain way. But your client's psychological freedom from EIPs' demands depends on recognizing their motives and refusing the EIP's often distorted, exaggerated emotional "reality." To help them keep a healthy distance and to preserve their boundaries and independent decision-making, share the steps below for resisting automatic reactivity to EIPs. If you like, you can print this out as a handout for your clients at http://www.newharbinger.com/53592.

Resisting Reactivity Through EI Awareness

- **No unrealistic goals.** You will get reactive if you set a goal of improving your *relationship* with the EIP. Instead, pick the goal of single successful *interaction* around a specific topic.

- **Stay in touch with yourself.** Your connection with yourself is primary. Even if you can't speak up, at least know your feelings and opinions apart from their pressure.

- **Detach, detach, detach.** Don't accept the pressure to get as upset as they are. You don't have to absorb their chaotic feelings and disturb yourself. Stay objective. What are the facts?

- **Spot emotional coercions.** Is their distress a way to force you to comply? Stay rational and keep clear about whose responsibility the problem really is. Do you really have an obligation to do what they want?

- **Channel your inner scientist.** Imagine you are a scientific anthropologist narrating notes to yourself on these interesting human behaviors and interpersonal maneuvers. You are there to observe and mentally label the dynamics, not react to them.

- **Don't accept any roles.** Don't get drawn into the drama by picking sides or playing the rescuer. Give yourself time to think and don't commit to anything in the heat of the moment, *especially* when the EIP demands a quick response from you.

- **Do they want your help, or your sacrifice?** Notice if your empathy or sympathy helps. Are they asking for your support or expecting you to make the problem go away, with no effort from them? An adequately mature person would appreciate your empathy and become calmer; they wouldn't dump the problem on you and make you feel you should fix it for them.

Interactions with EIPs are more likely to be satisfying if your client stays focused on maintaining boundaries and not becoming reactive toward the EIP's egocentric behavior. On the other hand, attempts at improving the relationship are more likely to be highly frustrating to your client, since usually EIPs have no idea how to respond to your client's openness and attempts at communication—nor do they want to.

If the person gets through the event and remembers even *one* of these attitude shifts, they've officially started using a more active and intentional approach to these very difficult relationships.

EIPs' Interference with Self-Connection

As we mature psychologically, we develop a relationship with our inner world and sense of self. We listen to our own thoughts, pay attention to our feelings, and dialogue with our better judgment. This is how we end up with a personality of our own. But EIPs' opinions can get between us and our communications with our inner life and our true self. As all children do, we internalize our parents' voices which then demand to be heard even when we are by ourselves: these voices may no longer be real, yet they still speak to us with authority.

These adopted voices can take a long time to uproot; in the meantime, you can help your client catch them when they happen. Here are some examples of what you might say to your client about these unseen influences.

Problem: Internalized EIPs Interfere with Feelings

- You seem to have a pretty judgmental voice inside that's dismissing your real feelings.

- It's as if a part of you sees your emotional responses as exaggerated, unnecessary, or foolish. I can see how that could make it hard for you to connect to your feelings in a genuine way at times.

- Sometimes you sound more worried about what you "should" be feeling than what you really feel. Do you know what I mean?

- Can you listen for that self-critical voice and tell me what it's saying about your feelings right now? Do you think we could ask that critical part of you to step back for a few minutes so you can explore how you really feel? (Schwartz, 1995)

Problem: EIPs Interfere with Reality Perception

- It must be hard to tell what's going on at times when [your EIP] gets so upset and starts blaming others for all their problems.

- Many people find it hard to hold on to their sense of reality when an intense person insists on their distorted viewpoint. When this happens to you, do you think you could go deep within yourself and reconnect with what you *know* happened?

Problem: EIPs Interfere with Self-Connection

- When others confuse you about what you feel and how you see things, you can start second-guessing yourself. When [your EIP] insists that you see things their way, it's easy to lose connection with your true self. You might even not hear that still, small voice inside you that tells you what's true (Gibson, 2000).

- But what if you trusted yourself and pretended that you *do* know? What do your energy and inner compass tell you? Do you feel good about what they're proposing, or are you dreading it? Let's take a moment to connect back up with yourself so you can see what your true self wants and why.

Why EIPs Are So Convincing

EIPs have this huge impact on others because as human beings evolved, they relied on other people's reactions as an extended network of vigilance. Feelings flash through crowds because it's the fastest way of alerting everyone at once if there's danger nearby. This *emotional contagion* (Hatfield et al., 1994) has served us well at a survival level, but it can be misleading and destructive if an impulsive, emotionally immature person is leading the pack.

An EI person not only says what they think, they say it in such a way that it sounds like the only way it could possibly be. That's their left-brained conviction about certainty: they defend their convictions regardless of evidence, and don't allow for what they might not know. EIPs stay away from self-reflection and big-picture awareness because too much information threatens their carefully curated security and self-esteem.

We all use psychological defenses to protect our security and self-esteem, but adequately emotionally mature people don't engage in the level of distortion and denial that EIPs do. Let's take a look at how the EIP's psychological defenses make them act in relationships and how that might affect your client.

Emotionally Immature Coping Mechanisms and Primitive Defenses

A psychological defense—or coping mechanism—is an automatic, unconscious, and involuntary protection against anxiety (Freud, S., 1894/2013; Freud, A., 1936/2018; Vaillant, G. E., 2000). The purpose of coping mechanisms is to help us maintain a state of comfortable homeostasis emotionally and psychologically, so we don't get overwhelmed, panic, fall to pieces, or feel threatened in our self-esteem.

Psychological defenses are the mind's reflexive way of shrinking an unpleasant reality into terms a person can tolerate, while avoiding or distorting information that is too distressing to accept. Our defenses are instantaneous, buffering against truths and emotions that might otherwise feel disorganizing or even devastating. It is important for ACEIPs to understand the automaticity and compulsiveness of psychological defenses, so they don't fall for someone's defensiveness as objective truth.

The maturity of a defense or coping mechanism is the degree to which it can take objective reality and other people's experiences into account. The immaturity of a defense is determined by the degree to which a person tries to alter reality, deny facts, or dismiss other people to make themselves feel better.

Like young children, EIPs don't deal well with stressful situations. Such circumstances are too scary or hurt their feelings too much. They can no more deal with strong emotional pain or fear than you or I could keep our hand on a hot stove. They reflexively flinch away from anything that feels too big to handle while simultaneously substituting their own view of reality, insisting that it's true.

For instance, EIPs might tune out unwanted information with the defense of *denial*, an effective blanket defense that stops the upsetting input from even registering consciously. For example, a person might instantly stop processing input at the first sign of bad news, later acting as if they'd never been told. Or they might go numb and zone out through the coping mechanism of *dissociation*, physically hearing the news but separating themselves from an unbearable reality by splitting their consciousness so things don't feel real. Or instead of taking responsibility for their own misbehavior, they might use *projection* and accuse others of what they themselves felt or did.

These immature coping mechanisms can seem absurd or incomprehensible to your ACEIP client because it looks like the EIP is lying or willfully pretending that a difficult reality doesn't exist. It's hard for the ACEIP to believe that their otherwise grown-up parent (or other EIP) could protect themselves with such transparently distorted maneuvers. But many times, the EIP's emotional immaturity limits them to juvenile emotional defenses against unpleasant or unbearable adult realities.

──────── Bonnie's Story ────────

My client Bonnie decided to temporarily cut off contact with her controlling and intrusive mother after her mother refused to apologize for deeply embarrassing Bonnie at a family dinner. After requesting space from her mother, Bonnie couldn't understand why her mother continued to email her with protestations of love and requests for phone calls. She had been perfectly clear about her need for distance and wasn't planning on changing her mind. Why was her mother acting like nothing had happened?

Bonnie was trying to understand her mother's behavior as if she were a mature, reasonable adult. But when we considered her mother's long history of emotional immaturity, Bonnie was able to see things differently. We understood her mother's insistent behavior as a form of denial: Bonnie's mother told herself she didn't do anything wrong, saw no need to apologize, and therefore believed that Bonnie couldn't be serious about no contact. When Bonnie didn't relent, her mother then projected all the blame onto Bonnie and sent emails about how cruel and heartless Bonnie was being for no good reason.

The less mature a person is, the more their defenses will alter their perception of reality to make it more manageable (Vaillant, G. E., 1977, 1993). In Bonnie's mother's mind, her denial kept her from seeing her part in the problem, so Bonnie's request for a time-out from communication didn't make sense to her. Bonnie's mother had reconfigured reality to fit her *feelings*; she *felt* victimized, therefore she was the victimized party and Bonnie was the one who was out of line.

When people are more emotionally mature than Bonnie's mother, they have coping mechanisms that help them deal with such issues directly and realistically. They can accept what is really going on while seeking remedial actions that mend fences rather than mowing them down. For example, by using more mature coping mechanisms of taking responsibility, respecting an adult child's feelings, and apologizing, they could defuse the situation and lower tensions. But like so many EIPs, Bonnie's mother protected herself with child-like defenses that soothed her self-esteem yet made things worse by reconfiguring reality into something other than what it was.

The reality-altering defenses that very emotionally immature people use are very similar to the magical mindset of toddlers and preschoolers (Fraiberg, 1959/1987). Their view of the world is shaped by wishful thinking, fears, imagination, and emotion (e.g., "Monsters are under the bed—whatever I think is real"). They haven't developed enough maturity to see the difference between imagination and reasonable objectivity: they embrace their imaginings and feelings uncritically, meaning that all manner of untrue things seem real to them.

Involuntary Psychological Defenses

The fact that we humans have such a multitude of internal defenses designed solely to keep us feeling relatively safe and calm suggests that people are easily upset, extremely sensitive beings that require sweeping protective measures to stay on an even keel. From everything I've ever observed, keeping emotional balance requires near-constant adjusting, and EIPs are among the world's least capable when it comes to regulating their own internal state.

Defenses are formed reflexively, not chosen. One of the most important parts of your job as therapist is to help ACEIPs understand the involuntary, automatic, and intractable nature of people's defenses. The EI parent is not trying to drive them crazy—they may not even be intentionally disrespecting their wishes. They react defensively because early in life that's all they learned about dealing with difficult experiences.

But as their therapist, you can help your ACEIP client recognize and reject the EIPs defensive distortions. Engaging the client in a questioning process is a good first step toward thinking for themselves ("Does that seem true to you?"; "Do you get to have your own point of view, or does being a good person mean that you must agree with everything they think?"; "What might you like to say to them if it wouldn't get you in trouble?").

That doesn't mean that your ACEIP client should excuse egregious behavior because it's largely involuntary. Regardless of the reasons for the EIP's behavior, your client should evaluate what the effects are on them and then decide on their own limits for communications and contacts.

As their therapist, you're just trying to remove some confusion from the situation by helping the ACEIP see how very undeveloped and poorly adapted the EIP's coping really is, and why they seem to ignore or misunderstand your client's clear communications. You are helping your client to see that they are dealing with a grown adult who copes like a kid: if something hurts or scares them, they wish it away or refuse to deal with it.

Primitive Versus Mature Coping

The most immature defenses are based on denying or distorting reality, which, when you think about it, is ultimately going to make situations worse. On the other hand, adequately emotionally mature people automatically use more skillful automatic defenses (such as *humor* or *anticipation*) to ease thorny situations or to prepare for upcoming challenges. They might even respond to stress *altruistically*, feeling inspired to help others even as they go through their own hard times.

Adequately mature, adaptive coping looks for ways to take an unhappy reality and transform it into something meaningful. Sufficiently emotionally mature people don't insist that reality should change and give them what they want; instead, they change *their attitude* toward that reality in order to bring their best possible coping to the situation. The more emotionally mature person controls what they can (including themselves) and looks for a constructive way forward, while the less mature person keeps pressuring situations to change quickly so they can feel better. It's obvious which method is more likely to produce more success in real life situations.

But sometimes such fly-in-the-face-of-reality reactions create a kind of power of their own. *Primitive defenses can work temporarily.* For instance, let's consider history and remember that reality-distorting defenses can make a charismatic leader look like they have all the answers. Larger-than-life leaders (or even dominating family members) get away with denying reality because they create enough emotional leverage to make it seem like they can do no wrong. They pull off their reality distortions because their defenses make them believe it so absolutely themselves.

But reality doesn't offer endless possibilities for denial. At some point, reality just doesn't bend. An EIP's reality by proclamation finally will snap when they push it too far. History is full of ultimate defeats when leaders overdrew their resources or outstayed their welcome. At an individual level, divorces or legal action may be needed to put a stop to an EIP's grandiose acts of dominance and entitlement.

The Benefit to Your Client of Exposing EIP Distortions

Psychoeducation about immature coping styles helps to clear up the confusion that occurs when an EIP flat-out denies reality or lies about what happened. Adequately emotionally mature people just can't fathom that other people would bend facts to that extent. As you help your ACEIP client spot these distorted, immature, and entitled ways of coping, it frees them from taking an EIP's demands and complaints so seriously.

Remember Jackie from the beginning of chapter 2? As Jackie showed, it can be very difficult to accept a parent's limitations, but her new understanding of her mother's emotional immaturity helped her to realize that she didn't have to be overly emotionally involved with her mother in order to be a responsible daughter. Jackie reported, "I've learned not to feel obligated to call her as often. I'm realizing that my needs won't get met. Previously I thought that in order to be compassionate toward her, I had to make myself secondary." Now Jackie was realizing that she could still care about her mother while taking care of herself too.

Instead of an actual estrangement from her mother, Jackie decided to separate from all the extra effort she had been expending in trying to coax her mother into being a more interested mom ("Why am I giving so much energy to these people, when the rest of my life is so happy and good?").

ACEIP clients to own these new parts of their self-concept can be a challenge, but once they get the idea, they will enjoy the process of assimilating new aspects into their self-image.

5. **Speaking Up for Themselves** Accustomed to being overrun by EIPs' expectations, many ACEIPs have learned to be overly acquiescent and not tell you their preferences. In therapy, they may be agreeable to the point of having trouble stating their true preferences or not complaining about something in the therapy experience. An example would be if they brush off your apologies if you make a mistake or turn up late. Such moments in therapy give you the opportunity to explore their tendency to make others feel better before they've even figured out how they themselves feel. You're letting them know you want to know how they feel so you can respect their wishes.

Your job: Instead of accepting your client's graciousness at face value, wonder aloud if they might have had other, less polite feelings in the moment. If they admit to less than positive feelings about something between you, don't keep analyzing it. Just tell them you understand, you'd feel the same way, and apologize. Your goal is to facilitate a straightforward experience of their being able to speak any negative feelings frankly, especially to an authority figure. Later, you could get even more benefit by reflecting on your interaction and asking them how it felt to talk about that. You may be the first person who has expressed concern about what their niceness might be costing them in their relationships.

6. **Regaining Healthy Entitlement** EIPs don't recognize other people's individuality, choices, and personal boundaries as legitimate. They often make ACEIPs feel selfish or morally bad for having their own preferences. But a healthy entitlement to our individuality and basic human rights (United Nations, 1948) needs to be cultivated in order for us to hold our own in the adult world.

Your job: You'll be helping your ACEIP client feel a healthy self-respect and an entitlement to being treated considerately, so that it no longer feels normal to be overruled by EI demands and expectations.

7. **Integrating Hemispheric Perspectives** The goal of therapy is psychological integration and balance at all levels, especially between the two sides of our brains. Our left brains analyze, compute, and plan, and yet we still must use the feelings and insights of our right hemisphere to grasp the gist of something, attune to emotional realities, tap intuition, and come up with original ideas. Therapy should help ACEIPs develop *both* brain hemisphere perspectives and integrate them.

As therapists, our left hemisphere—which seeks to oversimplify things—may encourage us to find *the* tool, the *one* school of therapy, when what we really need is a Swiss Army multi-use tool of several psychotherapeutic approaches that are effective for different parts of a person's experience and problems. The integration of cognitive and emotional-experiential therapies can be hugely effective in working with ACEIPs.

Your job: The best psychotherapies help people develop and integrate optimal functioning on both sides of their brains. You'll be teaching ACEIPs how to trust and integrate the strengths of different aspects of their mind, and when each is more helpful.

Chapter Wrap-Up

People in relationships with EIPs will pay a psychological cost. EI relational patterns are characterized by emotional takeovers and distortion fields; emotional coercions of guilt, shame, fear, and self-doubt; and outright attack. Helping your client maintain maturity awareness keeps them from getting swept up in EI distortions and other psychological defense mechanisms that can separate the ACEIP from their feelings, reality sense, and self-connection. Cultural differences can support what looks like EI behavior, especially in terms of boundaries and individuality. The goals of psychotherapy with ACEIPs are rediscovering feelings, regaining the implicit sense of self, offering emotional attunement and connection, rebuilding the conscious self-concept, speaking up for oneself, regaining healthy entitlement, and integrating different brain hemisphere perspectives.

Keep in Mind

- Understanding EIPs' emotional takeovers and coercive maneuvers helps ACEIPs avoid reactivity and enmeshment, thus supporting self-awareness and self-connection.

- When ACEIPs understand how EIPs' primitive defenses work, they are better able to withstand an EIP's behavior and accusations without taking them to heart.

- Even with cultural differences, it's still reasonable for the ACEIP to ask parents to treat them with respect.

- Learning to speak up for oneself, rebuild one's self-concept, and claim healthy entitlement to having boundaries and preferences reconnects an ACEIP with their inner world and true self.

Chapter 4

Your Therapeutic Approach

In this chapter, we'll explore the ways your therapeutic approach, your conceptions of what therapy is for, and your professional sense of mission all affect your work with ACEIPs. The idea is to raise your awareness of how your own history, ideas, and motivations influence your work with ACEIP clients. Your self-reflection will improve your effectiveness in working with ACEIPs.

Why Do Psychotherapy?

Let's start with looking at why you wanted to be a therapist. Think of this exercise as taking a baseline. In a notebook, copy down the following prompts and finish them with your first thoughts. No need to labor over them or self-judge; just put down what seems honest.

- I want to help people with…

- The thing I enjoy most about doing therapy is…

- As a therapist, I see myself as a kind of…

- The thing I like least about being a therapist is…

- I'll be glad when I no longer have to…

- I think therapy is most helpful for…

- I think the most important overall goal of any therapy is to…

- My biggest hope for any client is that…

- The kind of client I enjoy working with most is…

- My least enjoyable client is a person who…

You may have been drawn to doing psychotherapy for many reasons. What has motivated and energized your sense of mission about being a psychotherapist? In your notebook or journal, write about when you first realized you wanted to pursue this career and what appealed to you about it. And what keeps you going in your work now?

You may also have had other, deeper reasons for deciding to make your livelihood from helping people with their problems. Were there more personal reasons why you were attracted to this career? The better you know yourself and your motivations, the more you can help others.

How You Conceptualize Therapy

Now let's look at why you think people come to therapy, your beliefs about how psychotherapy works, and what you want to offer your clients as their therapist. Copy the prompts below into a notebook and then give your best answers off the top of your head. Even though it might be hard to express these ideas explicitly, you are unconsciously reaffirming them every time you do therapy. I think it's important to *try* to put them into words so that you know—at a very basic level—where you're coming from as you interact with your clients.

- People come to psychotherapy because...

- Psychotherapy works by...

- The most important, helpful thing about therapy is...

- The best possible outcome from psychotherapy is...

- People improve when they...

- It's not good for people when they...

- I would like it if someone described me as a therapist as being...

- Therapists should always...

- Therapists should try not to...

- The three most important things for me to offer my client are...

Even though you'll be refining your answers throughout your career, I hope these prompts help clarify your approach toward your career, clients, and psychotherapy overall. You help your clients most when you are as clear as possible with yourself about your beliefs and intentions as a therapist. Hold on to these answers in your notebook so you can return to them.

What Is Your Therapeutic Mindset?

Learning how to work with ACEIPs will increase your overall effectiveness as a therapist because you will gain skill in working at the most elemental levels of a person's psychology, and at a sufficient depth. Many people seeking psychotherapy don't have emotional issues only; they also have existential issues concerning their life's meaning. They need a therapist who is in touch with the emotional and meaningful questions in life, comfortable with ambiguity, and understands the human heart and gives proper attention to the client's deepest concerns. In order to be someone to whom people are willing to entrust their whole selves, you must be interested in the entire nature of their existence, not just their immediate crisis.

There's nothing wrong with more technical and cognitively oriented therapies—I use them often. But many serious problems require a wise person who can work with a client's feelings and dilemmas in a sensitive, growth-oriented way that can help them find meaning and fulfillment in their struggles.

I believe there are two very different mindsets in psychotherapy for understanding life and people: I call these *data mind* and *deep mind*. A *data mind* approach is characterized by a task-oriented, targeted way of thinking that prizes efficiency, loves data, and favors psychotherapies that use specific techniques to achieve specific ends and measure progress along the way. Data-mind approaches conceptualize people as subjects of conditioning: as if they have received faulty programming or deficient software. The client's thinking, rather than their feeling, is the focus of these approaches. Cognitive behavioral therapy falls in this category.

A person's thought patterns are of course vastly influential in their adjustments and their happiness. Data mind's understanding of distorted cognitions can efficiently address unhelpful beliefs. Data-mind approaches are tremendously useful for all sorts of symptoms and issues, especially those that could benefit from behavioral therapy or cognitive restructuring. These approaches draw on the strengths of left-hemispheric brain functioning, which we discussed in chapter 2. In these therapies, problematic emotions are seen as responses to faulty thinking or as learned automatic reactions.

Evaluation is built into data-mind therapy approaches. Data mind tracks progress, and targets specific problems, looking for the quickest route to change. However, addressing problems in such a focused way strengthens the client's conscious mind while possibly overlooking less explicit feelings and thoughts—however significant these may be. Since there are many confusing experiences with EIPs that the ACEIP client might not yet be able to put into words, such an approach could have trouble getting to the heart of the matter.

This more mechanistic approach may also be too similar to the kind of regimented response some ACEIPs felt from their EI parents in childhood. It sees human beings as thinkers with problem thoughts that need to become more realistic and less distorted.

Data mind feels most helpful when it catches people's errors in thought and thereby takes self-created suffering out of their emotional experiences.

A big problem with mostly cognitive approaches is that you are taught how to deal with the thoughts each time they arise. You have to put together new reasonable, realistic thoughts to counteract the problem thoughts as they arise, and deliberately apply them (Ecker, 2024). For me, it can feel a little too effortful and after-the-fact. I'd rather explore and shift the underlying paradigms, unconscious narratives, and emotions, so that change is holistic, and the client is no longer triggered into unwanted reactions.

Data mind doesn't explore the deeper issues of meaning that pertain to ACEIPs, such as personal identity, developing selfhood, or relational trauma patterns beyond the reach of conscious thought. An ACEIP's therapist should have an emotional awareness that can resonate with their deepest experiences. Our minds are not purely driven by conscious thought—only the part that we're aware of at any given moment. For the more poignant work of discovering self, working through concerns about self-image, and easing painful feelings of shame and self-doubt, we need deep mind.

Deep mind is associated with our deeper feelings, intuitions, and instinctive guidance, as well as our empathic resonance with subtle, nonverbal interpersonal communication and emotional need. Many people refer to this as having "heart," but in terms of how it operates in life, I think it is more accurately described as a form of mind—in this case, what I have described as right-hemispheric with its close ties to our emotional limbic centers (McGilchrist, 2013, 2021).

Deep mind is concerned with love, meaning, values, relationships, and sense of self. It connects us with emotions, the soul, the sacred, and ineffable experiences like awe. It's the mind that we have as children, before we are taught to think in a more goal-directed way, and it's this mind that we increasingly channel as we mature from mere intellect into real wisdom. It's the source from which art and spirituality arose in human civilization; it's the seat of creative inspiration and our ability to integrate dissimilar thoughts into new gestalts. Deep mind quickly grasps emotional situations, reading people's facial expressions and body language. It is the mind that parent and child share as they harmonize and attune with one another, creating bonds of trust and love.

I think deep mind is where you want to be as a therapist for ACEIPs. If you're not attuned to deep mind and instead rely mostly on data mind's clinical goals, what happens to the unexplored issues of emotion, meaning, and self-realization in your client? If you prioritize data mind's goals in therapy, your ACEIP clients might correctly get the impression that you are primarily interested in the thoughts that can be analyzed and verbalized, not the nearly inexpressible ones that confuse them and make them feel bad about themselves. Plus, confining your therapeutic focus to working toward specific goals may distract you from relating to your client at an emotionally intimate level. It also may prevent you from noticing potential new goals that inevitably arise as a person grows. ACEIPs have already had too many experiences of people keeping things superficial and emotionally distant when they really needed to open up to someone.

Deep mind is broadly inclusive of information, which gives it an edge over focused, analytical data mind in noticing certain patterns. Because it deemphasizes evaluation, it makes people feel safe and accepted in their entirety (Porges, 2017). When you sit with a therapist in their deep mind, you can feel their interest in you as a whole person. They are wondering about you, trying to grasp your nature. You do not feel picked apart, diagnosed, or mapped out.

In advanced technological societies, data mind is favored; culturally, we are goal-oriented, information-gathering, and transactional. It's harder to find people, therapists included, who enjoy exploring deep-mind subjects. That's unfortunate because deep mind is where real connection happens.

In an ideal world, we'd all have good access to both minds. But if you had to define yourself by one or the other, which one has the most appeal for you? If you see yourself as a deep-mind thinker, the ACEIP treatment approach in this manual will probably fit you easily. Even if you are more of a data-mind therapist, expanding your techniques to include some deep-mind elements can make you even more effective.

In the next section, we'll explore another potential aspect of your therapy approach: how your own past with EIPs might influence your therapeutic stance toward your clients.

Are You an ACEIP Yourself?

Since ACEIPs develop early skills in emotionally supporting their EI parents, there are probably a lot of ACEIP therapists out there. The therapist who is an ACEIP probably started life unusually aware of and interested in the inner world of needs and feelings (Miller, 1981). They learned that their sensitivity gave them an easier relationship with their emotionally needy or reactive parent. Growing up with EI parents and choosing psychotherapy as a career are a natural fit: both are highly concerned with other people's states of mind and helping others be happier.

Children who may grow up to be ACEIP therapists instinctively want to keep their parent emotionally stabilized so they become the kind of self-sufficient child who never causes worry. They tend to be sensitive and perceptive with a strong altruistic streak—they feel it deeply when they see their parents unhappy. They may even create a *false-self* persona (Winnicott, 1989/2018) that prioritizes pleasing the parent. This early adaptation to a parent's emotional needs can facilitate becoming the kind of therapist people feel comfortable opening up to.

Often such children come up with a *healing fantasy* (Gibson, 2015) in which they dream of helping their parent feel better so that their parent can have a happier relationship with them. Of course, this is impossible for a child to do for an adult, but they keep trying anyway because it makes them feel empowered, and because they hope that one day the EI parent will want to have a more genuine, closer relationship.

Unfortunately, healing fantasies can fuel repeated emotional rescue attempts that can lead to burn-out and even depression. With EIPs, no matter how hard the ACEIP tries, they are left feeling like they can never measure up, never sacrifice selflessly enough, and never do enough to help that other person. Because such ACEIPs are convinced that making a special someone happy will be the key to their own fulfilment and freedom, they may continue to chase change in the other person—something they never had control over in the first place.

If you are a therapist with some ACEIP tendencies, you can easily feel like this about some of your therapy clients. You may keep believing that you are only one more intervention away from transforming them into a happier, healthier, more mature person, much as you might have wished for your EI parent. Or you might become so invested in their change that you lose the neutrality that gives them the room to decide for themselves how much they want to grow and change their lives. These are forms of *countertransference* (Freud & Jung, 1974)—reacting to your client as if they were a person from your past. (For more about countertransference, see Stefano, 2015.)

In summary, respect *your client's* level of aspiration. Your hopes for your client may outpace the level of change they want, and that's okay. You're not there to help your client be all that they can be, whether they want it or not. You're a consultant, guide, and supporter, but you're not their rescuer, and they don't have to live out the healing fantasy you have for them. You will have given them plenty if you've shown a friendly neutrality and encouraged them to have their own goals.

Therapist Boundaries and Neutrality

Most conventionally trained therapists keep strict boundaries between their personal lives and their relationships with clients to avoid conflicts of interest, maintain therapist privacy, and prevent dual relationships with clients. They are also trained in a professionally neutral stance that respects their client's choices, refraining from becoming reactive, impulsive, or judgmental toward them. These therapeutic ideals of therapeutic neutrality especially help ACEIP therapists because they codify boundaries that prevent therapists from getting overly emotionally invested or embroiled in the client's issues.

Without these rules of conduct, quite a few ACEIP therapists might burn themselves out by jumping heart-first into their clients' problems. Neutrality gives them the permission they need to maintain a healthy distance, allowing both therapist and client to maintain their separate individualities. It also clarifies to the ACEIP therapist that they are not responsible for the client's recovery; they are only responsible for helping within the limits of their role.

It is perfectly possible to care deeply for one's clients while still honoring the factual limits of the professional relationship. In fact, the constraints of professionalism provide a safe container and framework (Winnicott, 2002; Langs, 1978) for clients to be themselves and grow in their own way. Without these healthy limits and neutrality, therapists' interventions could be overly influenced by their own emotions and countertransference. Without a healthy professional distance, ACEIP therapists might also be especially vulnerable to *compassion fatigue* (Joinson, 1992). Too much compassion and over-identification with one's client can lead to emotional enmeshments that help no one.

The Drama Triangle and the Role of Rescuer

For an ACEIP therapist, one of the most common types of countertransference involving overidentification occurs when the therapist feels the urge to *rescue*. Emotionally immature relationship systems create *drama triangles* (Karpman, 1968), rather than emotionally sound, healthy relationships in which people are capable of both emotional intimacy and individuality. In a drama triangle, people relate to others in terms of roles: victims, aggressors, and rescuers. Relationship triangles are widespread in any system where people have interconnected lives. According to family therapist Murray Bowen (1978), a triangle of three people is the most naturally stable unit of interaction amongst people, as two people solidify their connection by talking about, or forming an alliance regarding, a third person.

The drama triangle is a special kind of triangular relationship system—it's the kind of conflictual relationship pattern we love to watch or read about in a movie or novel. The characters' emotions run high, misunderstandings and conflict abound, and betrayal is endemic. It's also the way EI people often conduct their relationships, and it reflects an over-simplified, black-and-white view of life, where people are seen one-dimensionally as good or bad.

In a drama triangle, the roles of victim, aggressor, or rescuer are also known as the innocent, the villain, and the hero. Such roles create propulsive plots in fiction, and strong emotional engagement. EI people especially are drawn to drama triangling: it allows them to blame others for problems and pain while protecting their own sense of innocence and self-esteem. EIPs tend to perceive themselves as victims and to either blame others as villainous, or assign them the burden of rescuing them. Even though from outside the triangle, it can look like the EIP is actually more of an aggressor than a victim at times, that won't be the way they see it.

The empathic ACEIP is drawn to the rescuer/hero role. They feel an empowering sense of mission in making other people's lives better and—until they spot the dynamic—they seldom hesitate to step in on someone's behalf. For sensitive ACEIP therapists, the rescuer role feels like a bespoke suit—it fits perfectly. However, it can radically undermine neutrality and threaten boundaries between therapist and client. If you get drawn into this role, you can allow or even co-create boundary violations even as your actions feel justified in that they're doing good. But it's never a good idea to lose your perspective, even in pursuit of a rescue effort, or to take responsibility for saving someone else by caring more about their distress than they do. You are their therapist, not their protector.

This leads us to a truism: *no good deed goes unpunished.* In the case of a dramatic triangle, those who take on the rescuer role are often surprised and hurt when the people they're trying to help don't seem to appreciate it. Sometimes when a rescuer attempts to get between a victim and their aggressor (or problem), they're interfering with a pattern that's being held in place by an underlying dependent bond that resists any effort to interfere with it. The rescuer naïvely expects to be appreciated for their concern and is shocked when they are not. Sometimes the warring people in the drama triangle will even regroup and form an alliance against the rescuer, now in the unwanted role of interloper/villain.

In some cases, the base of a drama triangle consists of an addicted "victim" and their substance or behavior. A rescuer attempts to save the victim by getting between them and their self-destructive behavior. This often results in the addicted person feeling even more attracted to their addictive behavior and seeing the rescuer as an uninvited force trying to control them. In addiction treatment circles, this urge to rescue is termed "co-dependency" (Beattie, 1987). Groups such as Al-Anon exist to help hopeful rescuers pull back into a more reasonable position of neutrality, instead of trying to fix or save the person.

Here, the "good deed" in the truism means an action that allows one to feel altruistic; they may not realize they're enacting a healing fantasy from long ago about wanting to fix suffering people in their own family. They may even neglect self-care in hopes that their selfless, altruistic acts will make others appreciate them. But in truth, no one is appreciated when they put the burden for appreciating themselves on other people.

Altruism, self-sacrifice, and rescues are real and good things in life *when they're done for their own sake.* People are genuinely altruistic at times, feeling moved to help others when they can't help themselves. Where would we be without those generous human impulses? However, if you come from an EIP-dominated background where help means confirming an EIPs' perceived entitlement to rescue, be careful. Emotionally immature relationship patterns can take over, causing you to fall into a self-denying pattern that isn't good for anybody.

You're likely to have clients—especially ACEIPs—who justifiably complain of being unappreciated for what they do. In these cases, your job as therapist can be to help them explore why they sought appreciation from such a hopelessly empty source in the first place, and how their interpersonal pattern might skew toward sacrificing their well-being for others. If you can stay out of a rescuer role with your client, and don't take on solving your client's problems for them, you will model realistic neutrality and show them how not to be overtaken by other people's self-induced crises.

Your Mission as an ACEIP Therapist

Even though you must respect the scope of recovery your client wants, you are also in the privileged position of being able to see more of your client's·potential than they currently realize. There's no harm in exploring more than they're technically asking for, *as long as they're showing interest.* I believe your meta-mission as a therapist with ACEIP clients can be to help them restart overdue personal growth and refresh their existential right to their own individuality. (For other rights that ACEIPs might also like to reclaim, see Appendix C.)

ACEIPs typically need help in building their self-knowledge, self-confidence, emotional self-awareness, and deep connection to their inner self. As you help them explore their emotional issues deeply, they start feeling secure enough in their own individuality to free themselves from the self-effacing mindset approved of by EI parents. As their therapist, you can promote healthier goals of dynamic growth and self-discovery, improving their vitality and purposefulness.

That's what we're learning to do in this book: looking at the special needs of ACEIP clients, empathically conceptualizing their key dilemmas, and helping them understand and respond effectively to EI behaviors. You'll be equipped to offer effective help to anyone whose confidence and connection to self has been negatively impacted by an EIP.

What You Can Offer ACEIP Clients

Unless they have already done some work exploring EI dynamics in their family, many ACEIP clients don't know what they're missing in their self-development: they've been too busy dealing with EIP reactivity in their lives. As their therapist, you'll share what healthy self-development looks like and how they can cultivate it. You'll help them understand the psychological impact of the EIPs in their lives and teach them how to protect themselves with anyone who's inhospitable to their individuality and genuine emotion.

To do all that, you will make sure that your client has a *neuroception of safety* (Porges, 2011; Porges & Porges, 2023) around you. You do this by accepting your client in their entirety, not pigeonholing them in a diagnosis. They'll feel your genuine interest in connecting with them person to person, as you treat them with kindness and respect.

You are in a unique position to help your clients define and achieve such deeper goals as: rebuilding their relationship with themselves, reinforcing their own psychological self-preservation, and developing reliable emotional resilience under stress. You are an advocate for their growth, and you help them experience their own worth directly rather than waiting on other people's judgments. Helping clients get unstuck from feelings of unworthiness, powerlessness, or fears of abandonment (Firman & Gila, 1997) is like setting innocent people free from jail: there was never any need for them to be so constrained. During their therapy with you, your ACEIP clients can come to appreciate themselves as complex, unique individuals, and to let go of judging themselves according to the moods of EIPs.

As an ACEIP therapist, you help your clients undo feelings of inadequacy while redirecting their efforts toward a realistic goal: self-development. You help them reconnect with their feelings and instincts, and to understand their symptoms as necessary and understandable attempts to handle childhood dilemmas. Together you make sense of their struggles, while exploring the new option of choosing their personal integrity over placating others.

As you get more skilled in this therapeutic approach, you'll become the kind of therapist everyone hopes to find. You know what people have gone through with the difficult people in their lives. You also know what fulfills people and are crystal clear about what's unhealthy for them. Your ability to look beneath the surface, listen for emotion, and support individuality and self-acceptance means you will never want for clients.

As you help your clients on their journey, they will inspire your own growth and development. As you grow psychologically over your therapy career, you'll deepen your skill in helping people who grew up with parents who couldn't relate to their core being.

The Overintellectualized Therapist

By the time we therapists have made it to graduate school, we have faith in our intellect and capacity to learn. We might be drawn to cut-and-dried, technique-oriented methods that make us feel competent faster. Regardless of career stage, such procedural cognitive, mindfulness-based, or structured behavioral approaches to therapy can be very appealing to more intellectually-oriented therapists.

These methods are often touted as evidence-based: their procedures are clearcut and operationalized enough to be quantified for research. The more cognitive approach also fits with the record-keeping requirements of treatment plans and the documentation of symptoms and progress. All these things matter, but they're not everything. While the drive to operationalize psychotherapy and give it a research base is understandable, it doesn't equip us so well to work with our clients' emotions, which are subjective and hard to quantify.

These quantifiable biases have an impact on psychotherapy with ACEIPs. Many ACEIPs have already learned to over-rely on their intellect and language-based rationality to navigate a life lacking in emotional connection and parental empathy. Focusing on cognitive therapy alone with such clients, we can inadvertently recreate their experience of their EI parents: technically being taken care of but feeling unseen and deprived of deep emotional connection. As a therapist, you don't want to emphasize intellectual and cognitive methods with ACEIPs to the point of exacerbating the emotional loneliness they've felt from an early age.

If we as therapists had issues with EI parents ourselves, we may also have learned to downplay feelings and over-rely on intellectualized methods that make us feel more confident and thus more secure. Just like our ACEIP clients, we may have found reliable emotional security through attaching to our own thinking instead of seeking comfort from others (Winnicott, 1989/2018; Corrigan & Gordon, 1995). If we find ourselves over-intellectualizing at times, perhaps due to growing up around people who avoided emotional intimacy, we can change that by getting whatever help we may need to become more comfortable with our clients' emotions.

Choosing Your Clients

As a psychotherapist, you have more choices than many professionals do about the kind of people you work with over the course of your career. However, at the beginning, you're limited in what's available to you, so be wary of developing a specialty by default. Be mindful of the long-term repercussions of your job choices. Many therapists get stuck in an area they don't really like because they gained experience there and were offered higher paying positions to stay in that specialty. I urge you to take what chances you can to switch it up early in your career, moving closer to your interests.

Since you will necessarily use both your personality and your heart in your work, pay attention to the sorts of clients you enjoy working with and with whom you feel you can be effective. Don't treat yourself like a cog in the machine. You can't fake interest or engagement in this work, so find a style of therapy you enjoy getting better and better at. You may have to build clinical experience in other areas but focus on the methods and populations that are most appealing to you as soon as you can. You will probably be doing this work for a long time, so seek clients and settings that give some energy back to you.

Is there a kind of client that you've never been comfortable working with? Think, in as much detail as you can, about this person—one who perhaps clashed with your values, personality style, or sensibilities, or whose demeanor was just difficult for you to relate to. Many therapists learn what kind of client they don't work well with during their internship, practicums, or period of licensing supervision, when beginning therapists are exposed to all kinds of clients in the spirit of preparing them to be a well-rounded therapist. Once past this training period, however, most therapists won't thrive when deliberately taking all comers or disciplining themselves to tolerate a wide variety of cases. Therapy is very emotionally demanding under any circumstances. You don't have a moral duty to make it even harder on yourself.

So when you come across types of clients that you don't enjoy, don't work well with, or dread seeing, pay attention to your reactions. If they were off-putting in the beginning, it may never get any better, no matter how much you work on your countertransference.

You're allowed to be both realistic and self-protective by working with the people whose problems interest you the most.

Since you're reading this book, you are likely drawn to working with ACEIPs. However, keep in mind that many ACEIP clients won't be self-identifying as such when they come to therapy: they may have no idea such a category even exists. They may present themselves as people with self-absorbed partners, or a difficult boss. Perhaps their parents abused substances, or they're dealing with a narcissistic or borderline family member. Remember, many different diagnosable disorders may show the cardinal signs of emotional immaturity, and emotional immaturity as a phenomenon is not limited to any particular diagnosis or absence thereof. Even people who seem normal and well-adjusted from a societal perspective may only show their emotional immaturity in their intimate relationships, or in regulating their emotions. Through your ability to understand their experiences with EIPs past and present, you'll be able to help any client involved with EI people learn how to protect and care for themselves while setting necessary boundaries.

Clarifying Your Own Theory of Human Nature

To help someone, you have to have a grasp on what's gone wrong. Your approach to therapy will be based on your personal theories of human nature and psychology. For example, I am forever grateful to psychodynamic and Jungian depth psychologies for teaching me there is more going on beneath the surface than it seems for anyone who comes for therapy. Exposure to psychoanalysis taught me that a client's inner resistances can oppose therapeutic progress just as forcefully as other parts want to grow. I learned that clients reveal a tremendous amount about themselves and their issues when they relate to you like someone from their past, since much of their behavior and intentions are rooted in childhood experiences. They demonstrate within the therapy relationship that their past is far from over.

Although these deep therapies allow important insights, I often don't find their methods to be effective or efficient enough for modern clients. For example, I was taught to let transferences develop, to interpret unconscious motives, and to try to remain as neutral as possible. But many clients today would find this approach dilatory, aloof, and impractical, so over time I developed a more active and interactive method.

As you conceptualize what's wrong for your client, you'll instinctively refer to *your* own beliefs about human nature. You'll rely on your training of course, but often you'll go with your gut. You may not be able to articulate exactly how you understand people and their motivations, but it's there and it will be guiding your therapy interventions, especially during tense moments. Whether it's conscious or not, most of us have our own ideas about what has to go wrong to make a person seek treatment. I think it helps to write down in a notebook what you think causes psychological symptoms. Getting to know your own assumptions over the course of your career promotes your growth as a therapist.

fantasies and emotional reactions, and must make a conscious effort to recognize them as countertransference and work them through instead of acting on them.

Consider countertransference whenever you notice yourself having strong reactions or judgments that deviate from your more or less neutral therapeutic stance. Neutrality allows you to see your client's point of view dispassionately so you can give them feedback with objectivity and empathy. (Absolute neutrality is not possible because we're fallible human beings, but it's something to strive for.)

However, there can be times when neutrality is *not* the goal, such as when a person is endangering themselves, showing self-destructive tendencies, intending to hurt themselves or someone else, or being abused. You also may eschew neutrality when you believe a client is about to make a decision that will make things worse for them. Ultimately, the client has the right to make their own mistakes in life, so we try hard to be reasonable and neutral, even when it's a struggle.

When you're finding yourself getting reactive to your client, it's time for consultations with a colleague and perhaps your own therapist to help extricate yourself from a cycle of reactivity. This is not just for beginners; it's true at every stage of your career. Some clients may need to be transferred to another therapist because we can't seem to be there for them in a therapeutic way. (Seeking supervision or a consultation in such cases can also help document that you have taken responsible steps to explore the problem before fulfilling your responsibility to help them find a different therapist.)

When you propose a change in therapists to your client, you don't have to confess to your countertransference or reactivity to the client—this would not be helpful or kind. You can frame it as a pragmatic changeover to someone who might better meet their needs. It may be that their initial problems seemed to be in your area of expertise, but now you are dealing with unforeseen issues that aren't your strong point professionally. Not every therapist will fit every client, and we have to be realistic about our limitations.

Projective Identification

However, sometimes our troubling feelings will arise not due to emotional incursions from our own pasts, but from our clients' disowned and projected emotions. No amount of self-analysis will reveal the source of these induced feelings because they are emanating from the client. This is *projective identification* (Ogden, 1982), a particularly indirect, hard-to-spot form of emotional communication common among emotionally immature clients. It's a basic human form of emotional communication involving acting out. Babies and children use it all the time when they act in ways that make their caregivers feel as bad as they do, prompting the adult to meet their needs.

In therapy, projective identification happens when a client has some very difficult feelings that are threatening to emerge. Instead of being able to deal with the feelings consciously, they dissociate from them and act in ways that get other people to experience these disowned feelings (Schore, 2022). Because they're not in touch with these separated feelings, they can't put them into consciousness, much less words. Instead, they unconsciously communicate them to you the only way they can, by getting you, the therapist, to feel them.

Whenever you as therapist become aware of a strong feeling you'd rather not have with a client, consider projective identification. It might be a sense of boundary violation, irritation, anger, irrational panic, or even sexual attraction. Whatever it is, it will feel compelling but impossible to address in a straightforward, adult way.

How does this happen? Although it can seem like a psychic mind-meld, it's more likely that in your attuned state you subliminally registered the client's micro-expressions and body language, mirrored the cues in your own body, and then experienced the client's unconscious, disowned feelings as your own.

Whenever you feel in the grip of such feelings, step back and ask yourself: *Might this client be giving me a taste of their own unmanageable or dissociated feelings?* Knowing about projective identification lets you consider the possibility that not all your feelings in a therapy session may be your own. It can take the discomfort out of some of your emotional reactions as a therapist and signal that your client may need your help with something they may not be aware of yet.

Once you identify what's happening, your first move in dealing with projective identification is to unhook yourself from the feeling as much as possible. These situations need to be contained and understood by you before anything can be addressed in therapy. If you suspect projective identification and treat it as an unconscious, dissociated communication from your client, you have the chance to read their unconscious communication and use it to help them.

This doesn't mean that you speak about it directly to the client. They usually have no idea they are engaging in a feeling so consciously foreign to them. They would probably feel shocked that you are having these feelings, or they might feel accused of doing something wrong. The more skillful response is to use the information to make inquiries.

For instance, you might notice that you are feeling increasingly exasperated with a client's demeanor. Instead of challenging them about it, you might wonder out loud if there's someone in their life who has been especially frustrating to them. Or, if such an inquiry doesn't seem appropriate, the feeling may have to remain at the level of information you can't use right away. In fact, you may never find a way to use this information therapeutically. But even just speculating to yourself that their feeling may have been induced in you as a covert communication from dissociated parts of them can help both of you. You get to wonder what these feelings might be telling you about your client at a deeper level. And your client gets to subliminally experience someone tolerating and experiencing their unwanted feelings without striking back.

When the client unwittingly induces their suppressed feeling in you, they subconsciously watch to see how you'll handle it. They unknowingly identify with your struggle to contain and deal with these unpleasant feelings, while secretly hoping you will be able to contain it without reacting against them. At an unconscious level, they also want—again, not consciously—to see if you will show them how to master these noxious feelings.

Unfortunately, if you are unaware of the possibility of projective identification, you might react to the client in ways that make them feel you don't like them or feel uneasy in their presence. Projective identification thus can be thought of as a secret bid for being understood, while keeping other people and one's own feelings at a distance.

Chapter Wrap-Up

In this chapter, we explored both how you conceptualize therapy and what kind of clients you want to work with. We explored whether you're more attuned to data-based, structured, and intellectual approaches, or perhaps prefer exploring deeper, more emotionally meaningful topics. Your preferences for type of client and therapy need to be respected, so you don't wear yourself out trying to do work you don't enjoy. We considered how being an ACEIP yourself can leave you as a therapist with a tendency to get reactive to drama triangles, and how, since right-brain to right-brain resonance between ACEIP clients and their therapists is essential to the feeling of real connection that these clients need, we have to be aware that sometimes words work against the deepest kind of connection. Skill in spotting and using countertransference or projective identification can help you navigate moments when your own unconscious issues get activated.

Keep in Mind

- Take good care of yourself by consciously curating your career direction and being discerning in your choice of clients.

- If you are an ACEIP yourself, be aware of the possibility of falling into a rescuer role in a drama triangle.

- ACEIPs believe their emotions are a nuisance to other people. You help them relate to their emotional life as interesting and worthy of attention, whether by explicitly exploring their feelings or sitting in companionable silence.

- Sitting with and containing your client's unbearable and projected feelings shows your client that dissociation doesn't have to be the only response to deep emotional pain.

Chapter 5

Reversing the Impacts of Emotionally Immature Parents

Recovering from the impacts of EI parents is what ACEIP treatment is all about. Your role in these clients' healing will involve assisting them in self-development, finding meaning, and acting on their own behalf. So how does this play out in actual psychotherapy? This chapter is about concentrating on reversing the EIP's impact, and what progress toward achieving these goals in therapy looks like.

In psychotherapy with ACEIPs, your ultimate goal is to undo the harmful psychological impacts of EI parents' egocentrism and poor empathy, freeing your client to pursue their own healthiest and happiest life. You will help them transform self-defeating attitudes learned from EI parents and move from living for others to living their own true-self life with genuine vitality and spontaneity.

To translate these goals into specific outcomes, you will help your client to:

- Understand and deflect the control, shaming, and domination of EIPs

- Reconnect clients with themselves and restart their interrupted self-discovery

- Open up a more genuine, emotionally spontaneous (right-brained) way of experiencing life

- Feel clear about who they are, what they think and feel, and whether someone is treating them with respect and consideration

- Build psychological complexity and stress tolerance by using both their intellect and emotion, drawing from both left- and right-brain hemispheres

- Raise the adaptive level of their coping mechanisms

- Help them become immune to exploitation in future EI-dominated interactions and relationships

Expanding an ACEIP's Self-Development

By deeply understanding the unique psychological impact of your ACEIP client's relationship with their EI parents, you will be prepared to help them recover and expand their self-development. This might seem to be a Herculean job, but it has a straightforward goal: to cultivate and support in your client an existential and emotional awareness of themselves as a psychologically real, autonomous individual (Anderson, 1995).

If you cultivate this awareness of their unique individuality and subjectivity (Shaw, 2014) while you're with them, you will be giving them a healing experience even when you can't think of what else to do. Such is the power of trying to see the real person beneath their role.

The Foundational Healing Approach

Having an existential awareness of your client means that you acknowledge their presence as a unique person having their own experience of being alive. They are not just a client, role, or character; they are really there and experiencing their aliveness just as you are. I know it seems odd to have to say that, but our modern life moves so quickly and efficiently that many of our encounters with people overlook subjectivity in favor of pragmatic transactions. Experiencing the realness of someone is the essence of what Martin Buber (1970) called the mutually honoring "I-Thou" relationship, the opposite of an objectified and dehumanizing "I-It" relationship. To be related to as an object instead of a real individual makes it impossible to feel a sense of true connection and existential security (Firman & Gila, 1997), just the sort of dismissal that an ACEIP has suffered from EIPs in their life.

How you relate to your client in a session can be fundamentally healing just by showing them that their thoughts and feelings—their deeper being—matter to you. Of course you have a responsibility to analyze, assess, and diagnose as part of your due diligence, but let that be one of your mental to-do channels, not your only mode of relating. We can do our clinical job and still make them feel safe and seen from the very beginning.

Pay attention to them in their particularity, and let their unique presence *affect* you. This is what one of my clients meant when she said in amazement, "You really *see* me." She could tell I was truly present and relating to her through emotional attunement. I was having a right-hemisphere experiencing of her whole being, not picking her apart in a left-hemisphere, clinically evaluative way. I was beholding her; not evaluating her. Your interest and efforts at understanding clients' experiences tell them more powerfully than words that their individuality matters. This is the foundation of healing the impact of EIPs on ACEIPs.

However, you matter too. Being emotionally receptive and present with people needs to be counterweighed with necessary role-limits and neutrality as a professional therapist. Setting healthy boundaries around yourself and your professionalism demonstrates emotional self-preservation to your ACEIP client. If you let yourself be pulled around too much by your own emotions (or your client's) without the ballast of dispassionate observation, it can lead to blurred boundaries and burnout. It's a balancing act that must be managed for your emotional health; clinical training should help you relate to someone authentically on multiple channels at once, being both altruistic *and* self-caring.

By honoring your ACEIP's individuality, you let them know you believe in their right to have a self of their own. You plant yourself squarely on the side of their becoming their own person. Unlike EIPs that they have been enmeshed with or dominated by, their independence is not something you're afraid of. You *want* them to develop their own self and know themselves deeply. You let them know you're interested and willing to be surprised along with them by whatever they might discover about themselves in therapy. You give them permission for self-care (Krystal, 1988/2009). As you approach them in these ways, your client will experience self-development in every interaction with you.

Stay in Your True Self to Connect with Their True Self

If you cultivate a balanced right-brain, left-brain mode, you'll stay in touch with both your emotions and clinical observations. By not being too intellectual and by relating from your true self as much as possible with your clients, you will be giving them a very rich interpersonal experience—so different from what they got with their EI parents—thereby helping to shrink the EIP's impact on your client's personality. EI parents commonly are not anchored in their own emotional experiences and existential awareness of being; therefore they can't give their children deep enough emotional connection and recognition of their individuality. So when you as therapist stay present in *your* inner sense of self as you establish emotional attunement and authenticity with your client, you show them how it's done.

Before you interact with your client, take a moment to get settled within your authentic self so that you're fully present and ready to attune to them. To start a good therapeutic relationship, temporarily suspend the analytical line of thinking and open yourself to discovering who is there in front of you. To do therapy from an embodied, true-self-led perspective (Schwartz, 2001), notice your breath, feel your embodiment, and sink into your inner depths. Deliberately connect with feelings of warmth, love, and presence. When you connect with your true presence like this, your client feels their healing begin.

I used to wonder why, when I felt most eager, positive, and charged up, I inevitably ended up feeling frustrated and let down by the quality of my therapy hours that day. It makes sense to me now because I can see how the hunter-high of left-brained hyperfocus would hurry me past emotional intimacy and urge me to "score" hits of insight with my clients. Then when my left hemisphere inevitably felt thwarted and couldn't force what it wanted to happen, I felt a little irritable and impatient.

But when I felt a little low or not quite well, I would often have the deepest, most productive sessions. I could meander into the moment with my client, content to let them lead. Out of that less focused mindset, I peacefully listened, as psychoanalyst Wilfred Bion (1967) recommended, "without memory or desire." In this more right-brained space, often tinged with a hint of melancholy, I was more deeply engaged and attuned—just what many ACEIPs missed in much of their childhoods.

To me, it makes sense that by tuning in more to our relationship-oriented and emotionally attuned right-hemisphere abilities, we are better able to help our clients discover their true self. It's important for you as a therapist to figure out which of your inner states seems most conducive to self-growth in psychotherapy clients, especially with regard to *how* you perceive them.

This self-awareness can help you as a therapist figure out why you might find yourself feeling bored, disconnected, or frustrated with a client in a session. Did your left brain take over and get frustrated with the slow pace and endless detail of getting to know someone really well? Did it try to steer you toward making the session "productive"? Notice when your analytical, goal-obsessed side is getting in the way of relating to your clients.

Offering Insight Through Metaphor

If you sense that you're feeling a little over-eager to interpret and "get to the point," drop back and re-access your right hemisphere. Do this by getting a little dreamy. Let your mind free-associate. Contemplate your client with curiosity and empathy. You might come up with a metaphor for what your client seems to be going through and share it with them. This lets them know you're trying to relate to them as *emotionally* accurately as possible. Share your metaphorical insight tentatively, with an invitation for correction, so that the focus remains on them (e.g., "You know, as you were talking, I found myself thinking of this book/this scene in a movie/this fairy tale/this story I heard…"). Notice their reaction. If they don't seem to click with it, you might ask in a casually interested way, "Is that like what you're going through? What would be a better metaphor?" Your interest is the very opposite of what they experienced with the EIPs in their life.

There's nothing wrong with wanting to be productive or having goals in psychotherapy. But human development is not linear or programmable. It's a little like parenting: you're providing the conditions and emotional nutrients for growth, but the client's unfolding personhood will determine when and how that will happen. You can help set the restorative process in motion, but the timetable is up to them.

Why EI Parents Can't Support Their Child's Self-Development

Emotionally immature people's incomplete self-development shows up in their rather superficial personalities, their vulnerability to impulsivity and stress, and their tendencies to rely on rigid beliefs and identities. They can't support their child's emerging selfhood because their own is unfinished. People without a solid sense of selfhood treat others as interchangeable resources and use them for the security they bring. We can see this in Jana's story.

————Jana's Story————

Jana's heavy-drinking EI younger sister, Elayna, had an incomplete sense of self. After her divorce she had convinced Jana that she wouldn't be able to function without her constant involvement. Jana, tired of being at Elayna's beck and call, asked for my help in becoming more individuated from her. Since Jana did have a relatively strong sense of self, she was able to gradually restructure a healthier, more defined adult relationship with her sister.

Jana was surprised when Elayna adjusted relatively quickly to their new distance, adopting two cats and finding a new boyfriend. Soon Jana was not hearing from her sister very much. From feeling she was the only thing holding Elayna together, Jana now felt her sister had moved on. She didn't know whether to feel hurt or relieved. She did feel amazed that she wasn't as crucial to her sister's survival as she thought.

Jana came to realize that their relationship had not been based in two real selves in a real relationship. Rather, Elayna needed someone to be there for her, but her incomplete sense of self made the person in that role somewhat interchangeable. It was eye-opening to Jana, to realize her sister needed someone or something to depend on, not an adult relationship between individuals.

Since being Elayna's more mature supporter had been a big part of Jana's self-concept, she felt natural grief over how her sister had moved on, even though she was relieved Elayna was less dependent on her. Now that she was not propping up Elayna's incomplete self, Jana was free to develop a fuller sense of self based on her own interests and needs, which she did.

Two Aspects of Self Development

We all have two experiences of self. One is the sense of self that we feel intuitively and implicitly as our internal "I" or "me" awareness. The other is our self-concept—how we more consciously define and describe our characteristics as a person.

Our deeper, more intuitive *sense of self* develops in the right-brain hemisphere (Devinsky, 2000; Schore, 2019), and gives us that embodied sense of who we are. This self is based in our earliest emotional relationships and forms the foundation of who we *feel* ourselves to be. Our *self-concept* is a more conscious, explicit, and objectified self-image, located more in our verbal left-brain hemisphere (McGilchrist, 2021; Schore, 2019). It is who we think we are—how we conceptualize ourselves in words—made up of the adjectives, qualities, and labels we have assigned to ourselves over the years. Often people preface descriptions of their self-concept by saying, "I'm the kind of person who…"

Combining these two aspects of self-knowing gives us the overall experience of individual identity we need to get along in the world. But emotionally immature parents can have a negative impact on both. They don't encourage their child's individuality and are more likely to promote submission and family enmeshment (Minuchin, 1974) than to help their children develop their sense of self and self-concept.

How EI Parents Impact Their Child's Sense of Self

At the beginning of life, nature seems to be on the baby's side. Survival requires that parents be available and supply whatever the baby needs. Babies express their physical and emotional needs in such urgent ways that adults usually do respond to them, with touch, warmth, holding, food, stimulating interactions, and physical care. Unlike emotional intimacy, the physical needs of a baby extract parental ministrations in a very concrete, direct way. While babies need interaction and sensitivity to their needs, they don't require the kind of complex empathy that EIPs do so poorly. Many EI parents are still able to give enough necessary physical and interactional care for the baby to survive and develop basic trust (Erikson, 1950/1963) and sense of self. Most of the ACEIPs I've worked with in outpatient treatment seem to have received adequate early care for secure-enough attachment, but later suffered from their caregivers' inadequate emotional connection and empathy.

When a baby grows into toddlerhood, they seek autonomy, and begin to defend their emerging selfhood, which creates new challenges to the parent's sensitivity toward the child. Despite toddlers' frequent use of the word "no," their desire for good relationships and emotional intimacy with their parents *increases*. They need their parent's empathic sensitivity to be their home-base as they explore more independence and sense of self. Unfortunately, EI parents have a hard time supporting their child's increasing need for independence while still remaining available when the child needs to come back and engage with the parent to emotionally "refuel" (Mahler et al., 1975).

Since EI parents easily get their feelings hurt about not coming first or being rejected, they may counter-react with coolness or rejection when the child tries to emotionally reattach after a burst of independent assertion. Such parents don't understand that the child's spurts of autonomy are not "willfulness" or rejection. Nor do they understand that welcoming their child back into close emotional connection after forays into individuality is vitally important to support their child's emerging sense of self and independence.

Having had such a parent, your ACEIP client has felt the negative relational impact of getting too independent or assertive. They may have learned that the more they get in touch with their sense of self, the more threatened their loved ones seem to feel.

As their therapist, pay attention to how robust your ACEIP client's sense of self seems to be. Do they have a hearty sense of who they are and what they're interested in? Or do they seem uncomfortable, unsure, or apologetic about their own preferences and tastes? Through your careful listening and respect for their individuality, you can help restart a process of self-discovery that was interrupted years ago by an insecure parent.

How EI Parents Impact Their Child's Self-Concept

As their children grow up, the EI parents look for signs of the child's becoming who the parent wants them to be. *People-pleasing* gains a foothold as EI parents teach their child that their worth rides on how happy they make other people.

EI parents tend to categorize their children simplistically, such as saying, "He's the brave one" or "She's my problem child." The child may then carry that label forward in their conscious self-concept. It can take quite a bit of investigating in therapy to expose these early foundations of a client's self-concept. The following questions can help your client uncover these labels.

Define Your Self-Concept

These questions help expose how clients were trained to think about themselves. If you'd like a printable list to give to your clients, go to http://www.newharbinger .com/53592.

- What was your role in your family?

- I was the kid most likely to…

- My mother thought I was…

- My father saw me as…

- My best quality is my ability to…

- I am different from my family because I…

- I see myself as…

- What I most like about myself is…

- What I am least happy with about myself is…

- I need to be more…

As their self-knowledge increases in therapy, encourage your client to add to their conscious self-concept. Over time, their sense of self will be increasingly well articulated and accurate as together you find the right words for newly discovered aspects of their self.

A Strong Sense of Self Builds Resilience

When things get tough, having an integrated, mature sense of self makes you feel that you can safely retreat within yourself. You can be on your own and still function adequately, even if you would prefer to be with others. You enjoy relationships yet stay connected with your own inner world.

Given their own underdeveloped sense of self, EI parents don't know how to support their child's emerging individuality. So for many ACEIPs, self-development has been a neglected area. Fortunately, therapy deepens a person's individuality by helping them think about their experiences and who they are, integrating these insights into a meaningful narrative (White, 2007) that builds confidence and strengthens their identity. As one person told me, "The more I do this work in therapy, the happier I am." This person was noticing the sense of well-being that accrues as we connect more with our true self over time. As she gained in self-awareness, she saw how insecure she used to feel when she *didn't* feel connected to herself.

It is evident to me that human beings require self-awareness and self-interest just as surely as we need other people and a sense of community. *Both* self-actualization and caring for others are crucial for flourishing; but it requires a harmonizing balance, and when we tilt too far toward one extreme—even for altruistic motives—it becomes bad for us.

The Trap of Altruism

ACEIPs can feel torn between who they are and who they think everyone else needs them to be. The impact of EI parents' demands, or neediness, has taught them that a good person lives for other people. Thus, ACEIPs may aspire to an impossible level of altruism and worry about being bad or unlovable if they aren't self-sacrificing enough. When they start getting back in touch with their own needs and aspirations, they can worry they're being selfish, disloyal, or betraying.

EI parents promote this selfless ideal in their children because it fits the parent's emotionally immature compulsion to make themselves the center of others' attention. Plus, the culture around them also can drive home the message that putting others first is the highest form of goodness and purpose in life.

Some of our best-known thinkers in spirituality and psychology, including Viktor Frankl (1959/2006) and many, many others, espouse the idea that a person's highest self-actualization, sense of purpose, and happiness ultimately come from a sense of unity with and care for others. From such honorable sources as Frankl, we learn that caring for others and thinking about humankind is the fullest expression of our humanity. This is promoted as such a basic truth that it would seem heretical to question it.

Yet this compassionate ideal *should* be questioned as a therapy goal, because if a person hasn't been supported in developing a healthy sense of entitlement to be themselves, such sweeping ideals of altruism can feel psychologically impossible and shaming. If someone already has a strong sense of their own individuality—and I think many of these altruistic thought-leaders probably did—then concern for others emerges naturally in a satisfying way. They may already be rich in self-realization and have plenty to give away. But for your ACEIP client, high aspirations toward putting others first can easily backfire, exhausting them and delaying their own full self-development.

Whatever the source, a high bar of altruism may feel uncomfortably close to the guilt-inducing expectations foisted on your ACEIP client by EI parents. It's difficult to find healthy meaning or gratification in putting others first when you've been emotionally coerced to do so since childhood.

Any child who was parentified (Dariotis et al., 2023)—serving as a parental helper, confidant, or caretaker—grew up under an enforced kind of altruism that didn't allow them to think *enough* about what they needed. They were expected to treat other people's needs as more important than their own self-care. By being expected to always put others first, the ACEIP likely not only felt drained, but *guilty* about feeling drained.

Altruism can bring meaning and strength to your life—*but only if you have been supported in finding your sense of self first.* You may have to help your ACEIP client remember that being an adult means making sure that you care adequately for yourself and procure enough of what you need to feel healthy and whole. You can't neglect your needs and still have energy for others.

People-Pleasing Is Common in ACEIPs

EI parents make their children feel that the parent's happiness and well-being depend on the child's efforts to please them. When this is learned at an early age, it can generalize to all relationships in the future. ACEIPs may fault themselves for being people-pleasers, but sometimes it's an involuntary, defensive behavior learned early in life and can be very hard to change. For a child, having an upset or displeased parent is the definition of insecurity. Many children learn that an attentive, apologetic, or placating attitude helps smooth out the rough spots. Soon it becomes automatic to figure out what the authority figure needs to feel good about themselves in the moment.

However, sometimes people-pleasing arises as a natural extension of an ACEIP's genuine empathy and altruism. Many ACEIPs seem to have been born with an innate inclination to put themselves in other people's shoes. If so, it must be recognized as a potentially beneficial instinct, as long as the ACEIP considers their needs as well.

————Thandi's Story————

For instance, my client Thandi criticized herself for being "phony" and "obsequious" with her boss. She told stories of automatically laughing at the boss's unfunny jokes or not speaking up when he said something she disagreed with. She felt weak and insincere, compelled to get along with him at the expense of her own self-respect.

Thandi beat herself up for behavior she'd learned early with EI parents. Her parents dominated her, and she never learned how to express her differing beliefs in ways that didn't humiliate the other person—ways that were both honest and kind. So, she erred on the side of not speaking up at all. She feared that if she disagreed with her boss, she might do it in a defensive or demeaning way, like her parents.

For a client like Thandi, the most basic problem is not that they don't speak up or that they try to please others; it's deeper than that. Thandi's issue was self-worth: *she didn't feel she was as important as the other person.* She also "knew" she wouldn't be heard if she expressed her thoughts. The therapeutically important questions for Thandi were existential: Who was she on this earth? Was she as important as the next person? Did her ideas count, and did she have the right to contribute to the discussion?

Breaking Away from People-Pleasing

Here are some ideas for helping clients with people-pleasing:

- Go to the heart of the matter. Frame your client's problem as not about being timid, but as unconsciously accepting an assigned role of less importance. Ask your client to consider existential questions of their self-worth and their right to contribute. Wonder with them about how they see their place in the world and whether they would like to change this view of themselves.

- Suggest that your client first imagine what they *wish* they could say, even if they don't speak up, then describe this to you.

- If your client wants to know how they could've handled a situation, first ask them to brainstorm *what* they could've said and *how* they could have said it. No matter what they come up with, praise the effort: imagining a more forthright response is hugely brave in itself.

- After they offer some ideas, speculate with them how they could hone their response (e.g., make it kinder, clearer, less defensive, etc.) to invite the other person's receptivity and collaboration. Encourage them to use their imagination and empathy for self-evaluation: "How do you think you would respond inside if *your* employee phrased it that way?" (Refrain from the moralistic "How would it make you feel if they said that to you?") Teach non-confrontational communication skills, or assign them as reading (see Ellison, 2016; Patterson et al., 2012; Rosenberg, 2015; Stone et al., 1999).

- Go with your client's natural desire not to give offense by suggesting ideas for non-aggressive prefacing (e.g., "Excuse me, but I was wondering…"; "Hmm, building on what you were just saying, what about…"; "You know, about that, I was just thinking…").

- Normalize your client's feelings of fear, awkwardness, ineloquence. Your implicit message to your client: *You can make amends later, if necessary, but don't stifle your voice just because you're worried about not saying it just right.*

Thandi was soft-spoken and polite, so I encouraged her to go with her strengths and raise her points in the tentative, questioning style that felt natural to her. She initially felt

Imagined Encounters There are even gentler ways of practicing more active responses to EIPs. Let's consider the *empty chair* technique that started in Gestalt therapy (Perls, 1969/1992), but is also found in the *imagined encounters* of emotion-focused therapy (Johnson, S. M., 2019). In this approach, you ask your client if they would be willing to do an imagined conversation with the person they're having trouble with. They may hesitate, fearing they have to give a performance and won't be any good at it. Introduce it like a game they cannot fail at, saying something like:

How would you feel about doing an imagined encounter with this person? It's just pretend, but it's a good technique to practice expressing your true feelings. Let me explain it to you and see if you'd be willing to try it. We'll pretend the person has agreed to come in and hear about how they've affected you. It's like they really *want to hear the truth, and will be receptive to whatever you say. They won't interrupt you or argue with you; they're just ready to hear the truth. In this kind of situation, would you be willing to tell them how you feel?*

If they're willing, however reluctantly, you can say: "*Okay, so now see them in that chair. Picture them really vividly and try to get a sense of their presence. Got it? Okay. Tell them what you want them to know.*"

Typically the client will first try to address you, talking about the imagined listener in the third person. Gesture confidently toward the chair and eagerly redirect them, like you can't wait to hear what they're going to say: "*Tell it to them.*" You can use prompts like "*Tell them how it made you feel,*" or "*Explain what that did to you.*" Along the way, encourage them by showing your engagement in the imagined encounter: "*They're ready to listen. Show them how this has affected you. Don't hold back, they really want to know!*"

Notice that at the outset of this exercise, you have carefully set up all the conditions for a *positive* experience. (You can always do a more confrontational role-play practice session another time if desired.) This is not a high-anxiety practice session, complete with imagined opposition and frustrations; you are giving your client a safe atmosphere in which to experience the self-efficacy of getting through to someone, and in doing so perhaps satisfying a little of their need and wish to be finally heard.

When the person seems to have said everything they wanted to, ask if there's anything else. If not, ask them to take a few moments to imagine that the person is sitting there quietly, really absorbing all they just said, and finally understanding what your client has felt. (Even though imaginary, this can feel quite healing to your client.)

Next, ask your client to conclude with their listener by making a statement of their intention for any *future* interactions with the person. For example: "*And so now, [person's name], I want you to know that if you do this again in the future, I plan to…[insert intention].*"

This brings your client back to the present and gets them to think actively about what they intend to do now that they've finally been able to say all they wanted to. What will be their active, self-preserving response going forward? Since you've just activated their emotions toward the person, this is a perfect time to think about what they could do in the future that would make them feel self-protected and more in control of their own life.

Finally, invite your client to sincerely thank the person for being willing to come in and listen. Just like in a real conversation, you conclude the communication respectfully.

Writing to the EIP Perhaps the least scary way to communicate honestly with an EIP is through *a letter, text, or email,* which may or may not ever be sent. This way your client can take time to get their thoughts out without being interrupted, or worrying that the other person is getting impatient, offended, or has stopped listening. They can find the right words that express what they want the EIP to know, even if the EIP's no longer living. Written expression brings a unique sense of empowerment and closure, even if your client never sends it. (If you'd like a general writing exercise handout for your clients, go to http://www.newharbinger.com/53592.)

Reading Bill of Rights You can also invite your client to read aloud the ACEIP's Bill of Rights (Gibson, 2019), found in Appendix C or in printable handout form online at http://www.newharbinger.com/53592. Ask your client what happens to their energy and anxiety levels as they read each one. Sometimes just trying on the thoughts in that Bill of Rights can be revitalizing. There are usually a number of ideas there that ACEIPs have never considered before.

Identifying their Role-Self Your client might also be helped by describing in detail, or writing it down, what *role they have had to act out in their relationship* with the EIPs in their life. Who did they have to become in order to be accepted, or avoid conflict? Have them tell you what this *survival personality* (Firman & Gila, 1997) or this *false self* (Winnicott, 1989/2018) is like. How is it similar to or different from their true self? In what ways would they like to be more authentic?

Next, encourage your client to notice when their urge to play the role-self starts to take over. They don't have to change anything right away. Noticing the urge simply helps them see an automatic survival behavior for what it is and get a little distance from it. Later, you could ask them if there is anything about this false role-self they might want to be free of, or certain expectations they want to stop going along with. The point is to break down the role-self into smaller elements so that your client can begin to control when they use it.

Some clients might find that some parts of their role-self have served them well, even though it started out as a defense. That's fine too. The point is for your client's behavior to feel freely chosen and to their own benefit. If some social adaptations have made your client's life easier, they might decide to keep them.

Planning a reward If your client is dreading a necessary encounter with their EIP, suggest they plan a reward to look forward to afterward. If it seems silly, like they shouldn't need a bribe to have an adult conversation, remind them that dealing with EIPs is hard work. Rewarding oneself with something fun, affordable, and even slightly decadent can be an essential aid to solidifying new behaviors.

Supporting Your Client's More Active Responses

Despite all that I've written above, sometimes clients *want* to openly challenge and try to get through to the EIP in their life. They don't want to just manage things; they want to grapple with the relationship in a forthright way. This is all to the good, because actively confronting EI behavior overcomes all Four Horsemen of Self-defeat at once. I never discourage people from confronting their EIP (unless I think it could be dangerous) because moving out of the self-inhibiting and self-defeating passivity mindset can be so worth it.

Practicing Self-Expression in Real Life

In this approach, your client plainly tells the EIP what they feel and think, enjoys speaking their truth, and doesn't fret over the EIP's response. They express themselves in a clear, honest, intimate way, then let go of the outcome. While being understood is not under their control, the freedom to speak up is. It is the very opposite of passivity, immobilization, dissociation, and learned helplessness.

One day, if your client is feeling brave, they might decide to speak out and be totally honest and transparent with their EIP. I've had this happen naturally and spontaneously with several ACEIPs once they got totally fed up with walking on eggshells and people-pleasing. Being candid and honest can seem nearly impossible at first, but after a while it becomes the simplest way to proceed with such difficult people. If your client is game, they would simply experiment with telling the EIP politely and repeatedly what they prefer and practice feeling okay when the EIP doesn't like it or tells them they're crazy, disrespectful, cruel, etc.

Reexamining ACEIPs' Relationship Expectations

Growing up with an EI parent can accustom a person to expect and accept certain kinds of undesirable interactions and treatment. Many ACEIPs reprise childhood roles and expectations in their adult connections because they see it as the price of a relationship. It feels normal to:

- feel emotionally lonely

- feel like they have to struggle for attention and respect

- feel bad about themselves, as unworthy or unlovable

- see others as more important and more in need than themselves

- feel like they're never enough, that they never do enough

- feel confused about the legitimacy of their opinions and perceptions

- observe themselves critically, judging what they say and do

- let others cross their boundaries in an entitled way

- feel morally obligated to give whatever others expect from them

- expect relationships to require vigilance and hard work

Helping your client reexamine such expectations can reveal their unconscious assumptions, enabling them to do things differently in the future. If you like, you can print this list out as a handout for your clients at http://www.newharbinger.com/53592.

The Existential Impact of Having EI Parents

EI parents impact their children's development in day-to-day living, but I believe there are larger existential effects. The *existential impact* of a relationship is what one person's behaviors make another person feel about the nature, purpose, and meaning of life. Some parents are so self-preoccupied—or even cruel—that they foster hopelessness and low self-esteem in their children, depriving life of meaning and connection. Ask your client to help you make explicit the underlying *existential messages* about life they may have gotten in childhood.

Our early relationships affect how we regard ourselves in relation to the world. A parent's responsiveness early in life shows us what we expect from the world later in life: do we trust that things will work out, or do we expect to be let down and feel powerless? The EI parent has no idea that in dismissing their child's feelings they're having an alienating or demoralizing effect on their child. But they are.

If the meaning of life feels to you like something that should be left to religion and philosophy, keep in mind that our sense of *meaning* in life starts from the *emotional* roots of our earliest connections (Dowds, 2021). Life philosophies are not primarily intellectual or cognitive; they are embodied beliefs about what matters to us. Meaning is one of those right-hemisphere experiences that is as essential for emotional health as it is ineffable.

Meaningfulness is derived from what matters in life, and it comes from our deepest emotional motivations. So when an EI parent acts like your feelings or inner experiences don't matter or have meaning for them, it's like they're saying that *you* don't matter to them. That's a hard thing to recover from. Because of their own deficits, it just doesn't occur to an EIP that what's meaningful to them might not be meaningful to everyone. They can't see how devaluing what their child finds meaningful could be so destructive.

We all have a tacit understanding—or philosophy—about what our experiences mean and what these experiences bring to our lives, even if we don't think to articulate it. When a person's underlying meaning involves beliefs like "I don't matter to other people" or "I can't be myself," life feels pointless and depression can take over.

Your Existential Job as an ACEIP Therapist

Underlying existential issues about meaning and what matters are always present in a therapy with any depth. When doing so fits the tone, ask your ACEIP client what gives meaning to their life, what gives them energy, and what's important to them. Eliciting their thoughts about what's important to them helps them get to know themselves at this deeper level. You may be the first person to ever listen to them in this way. As you build your therapeutic relationship with your client, your understanding and emotional connection will make their inner world feel much more meaningful to them. As you try to get to know them, they will become even more interested in understanding themselves.

————Neisha's Story————

My client Neisha used to start her sessions with rundowns of her week, rarely offering any real feelings. But after I kept zeroing in on deeper questions about her thoughts and feelings, she began starting sessions by jumping right in with what she had been thinking and feeling that week. She finally believed that I was interested in what she was learning about herself. Her sessions went from monotonous to meaningful as soon as she believed that her growth and self-discovery were highly interesting to me.

As you get know your clients very deeply, you can translate to them what you have learned about them. When you simply say, "You are an exceptionally caring person who really wants to help people feel better," or, "Yes, when someone gives you the cold shoulder, that really shakes your self-confidence," they see their truth reflected on your face, and hear it defined by your observations. They understand themselves more deeply because you made the effort to know them well.

When someone wants to get to know you at a deep level, you feel *existentially meaningful*. Clients don't need you to write a philosophical treatise on meaning; they just need to know that they matter (Wallace, 2023). As their therapist, your attention and interest over time strengthens their sense of self and the meaningfulness of their life. Importantly for ACEIPs, you are honoring their depths in a way that their EI parent just couldn't manage.

Chapter Wrap-Up

The goal of therapy with ACEIPs is to reverse the impact that EI parents have had on your client. Through your respect and warmth toward your clients, you help them restart their self-development, especially by relating to them in an empathic, right-brained way, strengthening both their sense of self and self-concept. People-pleasing and playing a role are classic ACEIP adaptations to dominant EIPs and contribute to the Four Horsemen of Self-Defeat: passivity, immobilization, dissociation, and learned helplessness. It helps ACEIP clients to practice more active approaches to coping with the EIPs in their lives, such as doing role plays, writing letters, and doing internal work on changing their healing fantasies and false self-adaptations. Finding the meaning of existence is a felt process, based on discovering your individuality, feeling that you matter, and making significant connections with people.

Keep in Mind

- As you recognize and support their individuality, your client will develop a more deeply held *sense of self*, with a more accurate *self-concept* built on improved self-awareness.

- When you raise existential questions about the meaning and purpose of life, your interest in your client's experience of these deep subjects encourages them to think deeply as they explore their own mind and feelings.

- People-pleasing is an understandable childhood form of self-preservation; and passivity isn't weakness but an adaptive response to being chronically overpowered.

- Don't expect your client to feel real self-confidence before they come to know and value themselves as a person worthy of connection and being listened to.

Chapter 6

Revising Self-Stories and Protecting Vitality

In this and the remaining chapters, we'll focus on therapy techniques from several different approaches. For ACEIPs, effective therapy needs to be emotionally centered and experientially oriented. Internalizer ACEIPs tend to over-rely on their thinking processes, trying to offset the emotional insecurity instilled by emotionally under-involved EI parents (Winnicott, 1989/2018; Corrigan & Gordon, 1995). So if you make cognitions and reasoning the mainstays of their treatment, it reinforces the idea that they will find their best safety inside their own heads, just as they may have in childhood. You'll have plenty of chances to use cognitive techniques (Beck, A. T., 1976; Beck, J. S., 2021) as needed within the context of emotionally and experientially centered ACEIP therapy, but they shouldn't be the foundational approach.

Think of therapy for ACEIPs as a reclamation project. We're trying to help our clients rediscover their original blueprint—their own self-narrative—for self-realization and vital living. One therapy method can't do justice to the complex targets of ACEIP recovery. We need to draw on multi-factored ideas to assist the person in self-actualizing, creating positive relationships, raising their energy, and pursuing interests. Pragmatism dictates integrating whatever personality theories and techniques are most able to take our clients where they need to go. I think the best approaches are eclectic and depth-oriented, and in this second half of the book, I'm going to share the main treatment modalities that have been most useful to my ACEIP clients.

Before we get started, however, I do want to emphasize that in no way are the following chapters a comprehensive summary of all the treatment techniques described; instead, I pulled out specific methods that I have found particularly useful for the special needs of ACEIPs. If you like what you read about these different modalities, I encourage you to get further training in their techniques, as they all have much more to offer than I can cover in this overview.

How do you know which methods are truly useful for a client? I think the proof shows up in how *readily* clients apply what they learn in therapy. It's an effective technique if your client takes it in easily and uses it frequently. The most useful approaches are easy to understand, fit real people, and yield results. If an approach works, clients will naturally start using it when tackling a problem. When they start using the language of these methods, you'll know they've internalized them as coping mechanisms and are well-equipped to keep growing on their own.

Reassessing the Self-Story and the Fate-Narrative

Psychologically, we are imaginary beings. By this, I mean we have imagined ourselves into our sense of identity, and we imagine others into the roles we expect from them. Just as architects dream up buildings and philosophers dream up theories, every human being gathers cues from the people around them and dreams up who they are.

In his book on the origins of human beings, *Sapiens*, Yuval Harari (2015) suggests that what sets human beings apart from all other animals is our ability to imagine and live comfortably in a world of abstract concepts. People form ideas and treat them as real, making new "things" and meaning out of thin air. Manipulating mental abstractions such as money, markets, careers, values, and ideals—to name just a few—gives us a tremendous advantage in being able to create fulfilling and sustainable lives. We make up thought systems and create new concepts to meet our needs, and our own abstractions are often more impactful on our lives than anything tangible in our environment.

What we can imagine for ourselves will guide what we can become. We all develop a self-image, conscious or not, and that self-image is embedded in a *self-story*, an inner narrative (White, 2007) about our expected role in life that says: *Here is who I am; Here is what you can expect from me.* We also create an other-centered version of identity: *Here is how I think other people see me.* There are many forces at work in our lives and identities—many of which we were never aware of—but whether we look for opportunities or withdraw with anxiety is largely dictated by how we feel about ourselves and what we see ourselves becoming.

The ACEIP client comes to you with an underlying self-image and self-story that are based on growing up around emotionally immature people. They have been taught that other people should be considered more important than they, that they are morally obligated to sacrifice for others and put them first, and that their wishes should yield to others. In their life narrative, the EIP often takes up so much room that your client feels like a supporting player in their own life, living to react to whatever the EIP's lead character does next. We want to build back the ACEIP client's self-efficacy and sense of self to the point where they recoup a life-story arc of their own.

Unfortunately, once formed, your client's self-stories function autonomously, and may not be verbalized or even consciously conceptualized. They may not be aware of their underlying self-story and might even disagree with it, because their conscious sense of themselves might seem very different to them.

Jamie's Story

Jamie was a very accomplished, well-educated ACEIP woman. From a low-income family, Jamie earned scholarships and followed the markers of success laid out in her field to reach the top of her profession, meticulously building social approval through achievement. However, when it came to relationships, social self-esteem, and expressing herself in new creative endeavors, she often felt insecure and anxious. With EI parents and humble beginnings, Jamie couldn't believe that she was truly worthy of being accepted by others, just as herself. As long as she was in a sanctioned role, she felt more comfortable and confident. But as she started self-actualizing in new creative pursuits, she became filled with self-doubt, fearing that she would soon be unmasked as an interloper and then rejected by others. She was coming uncomfortably close to showing the world her true self. And that true self had been invalidated in her family.

Jamie was haunted by an underlying narrative from childhood in which she was still the unwanted little girl with dysfunctional parents who convinced her she was a low-status underdog, just as they believed themselves to be. When she moved out from under the shelter of her conventional success and started going in a new direction based on her truest self, living more genuinely and creatively, it triggered her old self-story of inferiority and fears that being her true self would cause her to be rejected.

Undoing Inaccurate Self-Stories

Getting free of these early life stories about ourselves is not a simple matter of insight. Jamie had insight; she could explain the origins of her feelings, but that didn't do her any good when they took over. Feelings of low status and unworthiness could easily overrule her legitimate accomplishments, evaporating her self-respect and strengthening old narratives of someone who would never be accepted by others as an equal. During these episodes, Jamie felt sure she would always be an outcast. She had done the best she could, but this was the self-story she felt she'd been given while growing up without parental emotional support or social inclusion by the peers she admired.

Painful though it was, Jamie's story had helped her make sense of the world. It was an abstraction of her worst experiences, distilled into a tragic underestimation of herself. Once set, this imagined self-image was so powerful that it could not be changed by any evidence to the contrary, causing her to find proof of her outsider status at every opportunity—even if it had to be imagined.

Such is the power of our self-stories. They become *fate-narratives*, convincing us that this is our lot in life, now and in the future. Jamie's first step in recovery was to realize that her self-image was being hijacked by a deep childhood belief about her low worth. She had to back up, disengage, and observe this takeover, so that she didn't automatically let this story be her only perspective. After fully experiencing the painful underlying feelings, Jamie had to work on detaching from the old story, just as she had worked on detaching from her reactivity toward her unsupportive and self-preoccupied parents. (Later on, in chapter 10, we'll see how clients can confront their rational mind with their irrational schema in a way that automatically releases the previous false conclusion.)

Jamie was helped to see that a fearful childhood part of her mind emphasized these beliefs ("my family and I are inferior") whenever she was tempted to expand her life and sense of self. Perhaps this part was trying to protect her from potential humiliation, but the effect was to deprive her of a fuller, more gratifying life.

Jamie had that part of her mind whispering in her ear whenever she extended herself in a more original, authentic direction. After all, the old self-story had been part of her identity for a long time. But once she could see the story for what it was and question its belief-structure, she could begin to put together a more realistic view of herself as she was now. She gave the name "little Jamie" to that part of herself that felt so excluded, and while she was compassionate toward it, she started to reimagine a new way of thinking about herself. (We'll talk more about personality parts in chapter 8.)

We can't just make up a convincing feeling of being whatever we want, but we can see ourselves with new eyes and update our sense of identity to include all the adult characteristics and accomplishments that weren't a part of our lives in childhood, thereby widening our possibilities for the future.

Once your ACEIP client spells out the story about themselves that they put together early in life, they have a chance to question it and reconsider whether it still fits. Many ACEIPs are unwittingly continuing to live out their original childhood roles, but by helping your client to objectively describe their childhood role and identity in detail, while feeling the feelings that arise, you give them a chance to reconsider their past and redefine themselves in ways that better fit their adult self.

Once we start living a life that is in alignment with our actual interests and abilities, we feel less drained and more energized. That's because an updated self-story eliminates the constant internal friction between our true self and who we thought we had to be

(Gibson, 2000). Since EI parents are usually not very psychologically minded or interested in other people's inner experiences, they have trouble helping their children identify and take advantage of their best qualities. These parents seem to expect their children to stay in their family and community roles, not thinking much about their future development or self-discovery. Even if an EI parent seems invested in the child's future, such a future would have to be something that the parent can relate to. You can help your ACEIP client create their own adult narrative, using their inner guidance and self-awareness to create a vision of themselves that really fits them. As therapist, you might be their first mirror for this newly expanded self.

Supporting Vitality Affects

While we all want the amelioration of symptoms, we know a therapy is working when we see changes in a person's sense of energy and vitality. Regardless of our client's referring problem, we hope our therapy will support more positive *vitality affects* (Stern, 1985) that raise liveliness and energy. Vitality affects are not regular, discrete feelings per se; they are a person's experience of inner aliveness, the dynamic fluidity and changes in their felt sense across their moment-to-moment experiences. They are surges of sensation and shifting experiences that make us aware of being alive and moving through time. At their best, they bring rushes of delight, discovery, or inspiration. In depressed people, vitality affects may be slowed to the point of emptiness or lack of motivation.

The dynamic, changing nature of vitality affects is what you would expect from a person who is open to life in the moment, free to be themselves. (As we'll see later in this chapter, this is why freer thought associations and more subject changes herald improvement in therapy.) If your therapy work is increasing their inner experiences of feeling dynamic and alive, you're on the right track.

Self-Care to Give More Energy

Before you say anything to your client, ask yourself: *Will my comment lead them toward more life, energy, and vitality?* If you're not sure, pause until you can figure out how to say it in a way that encourages self-care and conjures constructive hope for a more rewarding future, even as you're offering them different ways to handle the situation.

Take for example a client who reports that they yelled at their child the week before and is feeling guilty about it. Instead of explaining that could be harmful—which they already know—lead them toward self-knowledge by saying that we need to understand why it happened as the best way of making it less likely to happen again. You might find out they weren't taking care of themselves and were on their last nerve, or that the real problem was that they were scared.

In such situations, one of the likeliest problems is that the client has not yet learned to read their body signals that they were on the verge of losing control. Perhaps they never received parental encouragement to do this kind of self-monitoring toward self-care (Krystal, 1988/2009). You could promote the idea that as they take better care of themselves and become more self-aware, they'll feel more in control. If they thought a quick, sharp response was necessary to maintain order, perhaps you could suggest that they don't have to have all the answers on the spot and could consider stepping away for a moment.

We give our clients hope that instead of just feeling bad about themselves, they can change by understanding the causes of their behavior. We build their hope and energy when we point out a constructive way forward, such as repairing the relationship with their child through apology and listening. You help them change their self-story from "I am a bad parent" to "I am a human being who makes mistakes, but I make amends and try to fix what I did." It's easy to see which self-story offers more hope, feelings of efficacy, and motivation toward constructive change.

Better Functioning or More Aliveness?

Do you know how to be with people in ways that raise their energy and make them feel there's hope for them? I bet you do. It's called thinking the best of someone or having faith in someone. When we receive the positive attention of someone who believes in us, it fans a spark inside us. We feel inspired and hopeful about our future, and we can imagine ourselves in a better place in life. We feel stronger, more in touch with ourselves, and more integrated inside.

Our goal as therapists is to increase our client's innate sense of self-worth, encouraging a life that has meaning to them, with interests that nourish and uplift them. Too often we therapists get left-brained tunnel-vision by fixating on symptoms and raising functioning. These are important, but we want people to finish therapy not just repaired, but on a path toward optimal enjoyment of life, love, and purpose.

Many ACEIPs seem successfully adapted to adult life because they have learned how to please others and conform to other people's agendas. Their deeper unhappiness is often less visible. In order to squeeze into EIPs' expectations, they may have shortchanged their self-development by disconnecting from their emotional awareness, disregarding their needs, and ignoring their deeper instincts and intuitions. Continuing to believe in outdated life-stories that suited their EIPs lowers the ceiling on what they think is possible for themselves and their vitality suffers.

Make Sure Their Inner World Is Prioritized

Due to their discomfort with emotional intimacy, EI parents make their children feel that their inner world of thoughts and feelings is not important and should be kept to themselves (Gibson, 2019). They do this by discounting their children's feelings, debunking imaginativeness, and dismissing intuitions. They are communicating to the child that their right-hemisphere creativity and imagination are worth less than the concrete goals sought by the left hemisphere. Tragically, this prompts the child to distance themselves from the liveliest, most flexible part of their intellectual capital—thereby shrinking their ability to come up with creative solutions and independent thinking.

Basically, EI parents give the message that *they* will evaluate whether their child's thoughts and feelings are worthwhile enough to warrant support or sympathy. ACEIPs' expectation of having their feelings *evaluated* rather than *responded to* shows every time they preface their statements with "This is such a small thing I'm embarrassed to say it" or "It's just that…" But when you point out this self-minimizing behavior to them, ACEIPs often don't get it at first. They think they're being realistic or politely humble in discounting their feelings and inner experiences.

When EI parents teach their children to devalue their inner world, this cements the parent's power to control the child psychologically. By undermining the legitimacy of their child's ideas and emotions, the parent's attitude dominates. But as your client becomes aware of how emotionally ignored or psychologically subjugated they felt, they might begin to question those parents' reactions.

Your role as therapist is to help your ACEIP client to reverse this early conditioning and once again trust that their inner experiences are worthy of being taken seriously.

Don't Let Things Stay Boring

ACEIPs sometimes report that their past therapists tended to over-focus on their obvious strengths and insights, implying that they were already doing pretty well. It was as if the therapist didn't feel they had anything else to offer such a high-functioning person. ACEIP clients often seem like they're already doing better than most people the therapist sees. But a therapist unaware of ACEIP dynamics can miss that the client's "good" functioning and independence *are* clinical signs of classic ACEIP maladaptations of putting the emotional needs of others first, while not meeting one's own. Often these clients unconsciously try to not be a bother and to stay in the therapist's good graces by not asking too much from them.

Sometimes therapists not knowledgeable about ACEIPs also can feel stumped because the sessions gradually become more and more superficial and boring. Such a therapist might describe feeling bored or disengaged and yet unable to think of how to deepen the session.

You can consider both of these situations as unconscious reenactments of the EI parent–ACEIP dynamic. As the ACEIP client gains familiarity with the therapist, they unconsciously begin to play out childhood patterns of trying to maintain connection with EI parents by becoming less and less trouble and showing fewer and fewer needs. They know that EI parents are terrified of emotional intimacy and unskilled in meeting emotional needs, so they unconsciously assume the therapist will be the same. They are protecting the relationship by showing only the superficiality and absence of need that they think earned their parent's approval.

On the therapist's side—especially if the therapist has an ACEIP history themselves—they may inadvertently let sessions slide into a comfortable routine where nothing much is demanded of the therapist or client, where dull, daily concerns are processed and reprocessed. The therapist might feel uncomfortable prompting more emotional intimacy or worry that they will seem rude or disinterested if they don't follow the client's conversational lead.

But many times, abrupt subject changes into deeper territory are a relief to both parties. For instance, you might ask things like the following:

- I can't help but wonder what's really on your mind today. Why don't you take a moment and let yourself drop down into something that you've been feeling lately.

- You sound like everything's going great, but I get the feeling there's more there.

- I wonder what you might need help with today.

- It could just be me, but it seems we're kind of staying on the surface of things today. Does it feel like that to you too?

- I'm hearing about what you've been doing, but not much about your feelings. What are you feeling right now, as you tell me about these things?

- Are you feeling like you're getting what you want out of the session so far today?

- You know, today I find myself wanting to hear about something that feels more emotional and alive for you. Do you know what I mean?

Often the client will confess that they really don't have much to say today, or don't know what to talk about. (Actually, they have their entire lives and their whole self to talk about, but they've been trained to consider that as unimportant.) Basically, they're saying, "Now that the immediate crisis has passed, I have no experience in taking things to a deeper level. So I guess I'll do my part and keep to safe topics."

Here's your chance to teach your ACEIP client how to take their inner world seriously and visit those underexplored parts of their mind, emotions, imagination, and intuitive

Find Their Boundaries

Having your boundaries transgressed is exhausting. It demands energy-draining self-control and stirs up emotional reactivity and stress. Since boundary transgression is a hallmark of emotionally immature behavior, your ACEIP client is likely to spend a lot of their energy on how to respond to EIPs who try their limits.

As a person gets better at noticing and accepting their true feelings and energy levels, they begin to feel more confident about the kind of boundaries they need. Your client can't set good personal boundaries until they can *feel* their reactions to other people's behavior—something that many ACEIPs are trained out of at an early age—so you at first may have to help them sense the discomfort that tells them where a boundary needs to be.

Boundaries might be external or internal. They might be limits your client places on other people's behavior (Tawwab, 2021), or internal boundaries against the unreasonable expectations your client puts on themselves. As their therapist, you will help them feel healthily entitled to setting comfortable limits and being treated respectfully—including by themselves. Simply asking a client to describe the fluctuations in their energy levels when they think certain thoughts will help them to tune in to a very reliable way of sensing a healthier direction. When the thought of something exhausts you, perhaps it's not good for you to do it—or at least not to do it in the same old pattern.

Change Beliefs and Thought Patterns

Using aspects of Coherence Therapy and related skills of memory reconsolidation (Ecker & Hulley, 1996, 2005–2019), which we will get to in chapter 10, you'll help your client clarify and change depleting beliefs, motives, and self-narratives that have been part of their story since childhood. You'll explore how their beliefs were shaped by frightening childhood experiences or fears of being disloyal or otherwise hurting their parents. You'll begin to see the self-preserving motives behind your client's symptomatic behavior. By listening carefully for underlying assumptions, you as therapist are going to help them winnow out the beliefs, motives, and life narratives (White, 2007) that may no longer fit their adult lives, and see if they are ready to release them.

Deal with Healing Fantasies, Grief, and Resentment

One of your clients' ongoing challenges will be their *healing fantasies*, which are based on the hope that one day their parent or other EIP finally will become a warm person who is capable of a close, empathic relationship. Although your client has grown up and started their own life, they may still feel outside approval is necessary to deserve happiness. As they mature in therapy and become more realistic about the slim chances of their EIP's changing, they also may become more accepting of what the actual relationship can offer them.

Often this acceptance will bring sadness and even grief, as the person realizes what a lost cause it can be to try to get their EIP to change against their will. They begin to feel how tiring it is to always put the EIP first. Once a client sees how much energy is lost in chasing the vision of an ideal parent or reformed EIP, they may find it easier to become increasingly realistic and self-protective around that person. By letting go of these old self-stories about how they should be able to improve the relationship, they gradually begin to release resentful attitudes and become more realistic about their EIP's limitations.

Assessing Your Client's Self-Development Progress

Long before I started focusing on emotional maturity and immaturity, I noticed how clients who were benefiting from therapy and getting in touch with their true self also started expressing themselves with more direction and vitality in our sessions. They stopped chatting at the beginning of their sessions and went straight into their therapeutic work. They no longer seemed indecisive or apologetic about their concerns. They seemed more spontaneous, changed topics fluidly, and talked readily about the meaning of their emotional experiences. They didn't try to stay on the surface or be socially correct; they were actively trying to figure things out. They showed increasing insight, excited by their improved understanding of what was *really* going on. These were signs of their integrative inner work, evidence they were drawing on right-brain holistic insights to increase the scope of their understanding.

Increased Metaphorical and Associational Thought

As my clients got more in touch with themselves, their vitality and interest in understanding themselves increased. They described their experiences in a way that deepened my empathy for them. I increasingly felt like I was really grasping what they were feeling. These were signs that their growth had moved us further into a harmonious state of right-brain to right-brain communication, that state of interpersonal neurological attunement that facilitates deep connections between people (Schore, 2019).

My improving clients also used more metaphorical speech. It was as though when they became more self-accepting and whole, they turned poetic. They naturally used metaphorical examples to capture and convey the *feeling tone* of their experiences. Their symbolic speech sparked emotional and aesthetic reactions and associations in me, deepening my comprehension. To me, their shift in communication style was very noticeable, catching my attention like a gold coin on the beach. When I reflected on this to my clients, they would invariably agree that they were feeling very in touch with themselves.

Also, their thoughts became more free-associational. They would spontaneously interrupt themselves when new thoughts crossed their mind, indicating we were on the cutting edge of their self-discovery. They seemed fully present in the moment as they tried to help me understand what it was like for them. Their energy seemed to flow along its own natural tributaries, instead of being artificially narrowed into a single line of thought. I've come to realize that when a client apologizes to you for being all over the map and not staying on one topic, that usually is a good sign that they have felt free to follow their own inspiration and vitality—in other words, to be themselves with you.

I always reassure clients that I enjoy their more freewheeling expression, find it very easy to follow them, and would speak up if I ever had any trouble understanding them. In this way, I am explicitly approving of their heightened spontaneity and increased vitality. ACEIPs often can't believe you aren't annoyed by their energetic mental hopping around, and they're surprised that you can keep up with them. Actually, it's never hard to keep up with a person when you're interested in what they're saying. But they grew up with impatient EIPs who had limited attention spans and expected them to get to the point quickly.

A Shift in Communication Style

Robert Langs, a psychoanalyst and psychotherapy researcher, studied how communication styles differ depending on a person's internal psychological capacities (Langs, 1978). The more open, symbolic, metaphorical speech that I described above is characteristic of what he calls *Type A communicators*. This type of client is often self-referred and has the capacity for insight and symbolic thought. They have the words to make their inside worlds accessible, stirring interest, empathy, and curiosity in their listener, reporting not only facts, but context and feelings too. It feels like their real self is talking. This style naturally supports interest and connection in a way that other communication styles do not.

I've found that when clients begin to shift into richer levels of Type A communication, it's a sign that they are on the right track and beginning to explore the depths of themselves. From a neurological perspective, Langs's Type A communication style seems to reflect a more integrated and right-brained processing style (McGilchrist, 2021; Schore, 2019). They show more empathy, a deeper sense of self, and their apt metaphors evoke emotional understanding in an embodied, authentic way. Increased use of symbolic communication suggests that the client is integrating both conceptual and experiential understanding—i.e., the kind of deep insight that changes a person.

I have had a number of clients who look back in humor on the early days of therapy when they hated imagery exercises and didn't know what I meant by a metaphor. It was hard for them to access that part of their mind at the beginning, but toward the end of their therapy, they were readily communicating in this symbolic speech to express their self-knowledge more deeply and to enhance our mutual understanding. Regaining Type A metaphorical self-expression is like restoring one's soul.

In Langs's system, *Type B communicators* are very different. They come to therapy communicating in what Langs calls an "action-discharge" style, where they dump their unsettled feelings into the therapist through projective identification, forcing them to contain and metabolize their distress. They don't seek to understand so much as to get rid of their feelings. Their communication is a spewing that doesn't lead to insight or growth. This is a style that is common among externalizers and emotionally immature people.

However, in both Types A and B, communication is still being attempted between people, whether through symbolic speech, blowing off steam, or through projective identification interactions. Even in Type B, there's an attempt toward some level of connection. But there's a third type, the *Type C communicator*, for whom language is not a bridge to connection. In fact, its flatness and absence of depth or substance is used as a *barrier* to connection. Langs describes how in Type C communications "…meaninglessness is the model, the lie is the mode, and deception is the goal" (Langs, 1978, p. 125)—perhaps to avoid a disorganizing chaotic anxiety that roils inside the core of a person. However, I reinterpret what Langs calls lying and deception as unconscious evasions aimed at defensive psychological preservation, not conscious manipulation. I consider Type C communicators to be an especially severe type of disconnected EIP.

My clients have often complained about the meaninglessness inherent in this type's communications. They describe *brain scramble* experiences, a term used by psychotherapist Jenny Walters to describe the confusion that comes from trying to deal with highly defensive, self-centered people. Real communication is often impossible because the Type C communicator is trying *not* to be known, to not go deeper into their inner experience or truth. Telling the truth to another person stirs emotional intimacy and this seems to threaten Type C EIPs, perhaps due to fears that their fragile sense of self could be annihilated through exposure.

This is exactly the extremely superficial, meaning-destroying communication that many of my clients have described as driving them crazy when trying to relate to their EIP. It seems like they should be able to communicate—after all, they're speaking the same language—but the EIP frustrates meaningful connection and communication at every turn. It can be a huge relief and revelation to your ACEIP client when you explain these communication dynamics and motivations to them.

What Does "Getting Better" Really Mean?

If you're not going to be repeatedly assessing your clients with symptom checklists, how do you tell when they're getting better? Changes start happening deep inside before the person shows changes in their behavior or symptoms. Being able to spot the improvements described below will help you recognize that your client is progressing.

Clients show more access to their inner world. As therapy progresses, you increasingly feel you're really getting to know the person. Instead of just reporting events, they offer insight into their feelings and thoughts during events. More specifically, the client's increasing use of *metaphor, imagery, descriptions of emotional experiences and insights,* and *Type A communications* are specific signs that the client is gaining in self-awareness and self-development. These trends toward livelier speech show that your client is reversing the impact of EI parents' inhibiting effect on their vitality. Their increased self-knowledge and confidence in their inner world reveal increased trust of their insights and intuitions.

Clients show a stronger sense of self. While this shift can be harder to pin down, you will begin to hear statements from your client that are more self-defined and self-expressive, especially those involving EIPs. For instance, they might say things that show self-awareness, like "It's just not the kind of person I am…;" "My feelings were really hurt;" or "It felt so right to me!" Or they might reveal self-preserving boundary instincts like indignation ("I couldn't believe they would say that to me!"), anger ("I got so mad"), distaste ("I actually felt queasy"), or limit-setting ("I told her if she kept telling me what to do, I would have to leave"). Such statements reveal that your clients feel themselves to be real individuals with their own identity and adult rights. Their interpersonal tone feels more assertive and definite, as though they are claiming the right to their existence.

Clients show decreased reactivity to EI behavior. Decreased reactivity to EIPs happens when emotional triggers in the brain have been worked through and underlying distorted beliefs that condone EIPs' domination have been rejected as false. When you help a client use detachment, observation, silent self-narration, and maintaining deliberate self-connection as they deal with EIPs, you are teaching them to respond from their thinking, observing minds instead of blindly reacting at an emotional level.

When your client has developed more of a sense of self and more self-confidence— with fewer distorted beliefs about what they owe other people—they will not feel as obliged to serve EIPs' needs. When your client no longer feels guilty about or ashamed of their own individuality and preferences, it won't matter to them so much whether or not EIPs give their blessings. When your client is clear about their right to create their own life and boundaries, they will no longer react defensively to EIPs' attempts to coerce and control them. They will just stop listening.

Clients start to show higher level coping mechanisms. Emotionally immature people, by definition, use different degrees of emotionally immature defenses or coping mechanisms, including denial (didn't happen), projection (someone else did it), and simplistic rationalization (I may have done it, but here's why it's okay), while ACEIPs often show more mid-range intellectualizing and rationalizing defenses that try to alter their own feelings and thoughts to conform to others' expectations. As clients grow in self-development and recover from the inhibitory impacts of EIPs, they start to show more effective, or mature, coping mechanisms as they deal with stress in their lives.

For instance, they are increasingly able to accept both internal and external reality on its own terms, without distorting circumstances or denying their own reactions. Some of these more mature psychological mechanisms include *altruism* ("I feel better when I help other people"); *humor* ("This is so funny"); *suppression* ("I'm not going to think about that right now"); *anticipation* ("This could happen if I do that"); and *sublimation* ("I channel my instincts into harmless competition, creativity, or esthetic appreciation") (Vaillant, G. E., 2000). Other more mature coping mechanisms might include *self-observation* ("Are my efforts working?"); *self-assertion* ("I'm going to try to change this situation to my benefit"); and *affiliation* ("I need some company to get through this"). At this level of coping, a person is putting their energy into dealing actively with a problematic situation on a very realistic level. They accept reality on its own terms and are energized by working at problem-solving.

Altruism is one mature coping mechanism I used to find a little harder to understand, as it seemed more like an elective behavior than a coping mechanism for stress and anxiety. I finally understood how it helps coping when talking to a friend whose father was undergoing treatment in the hospital. She told me how difficult the situation was, then spontaneously shared that she'd been thinking that when all this was over, she might sign up to read to or just visit elderly people in nursing homes. "They've lived through so much and have no one to talk to," she said. "It would be fascinating to hear their stories."

This person's altruistic fantasy seemed to energize her as she talked about it. That's the mark of a mature coping mechanism: not only does it lower our stress, but it actively shifts our focus to a constructive goal, improving our mood and prompting us to feel gratified and empowered. We can learn these more mature methods by being exposed to them in our relationships, and therapy is a great place to do that.

The most mature coping mechanisms are flexible and hardy, working against the entropy or "settling" that can happen after our first attempts at problem-solving don't work. When using the most mature coping mechanisms, people bring the best of both brain hemispheres to bear on challenging situations or fears. We can think and feel our way through a difficult reality if we're not trying to deny or alter it. More adaptive and creative coping mechanisms handle stress in adaptive ways that aren't draining.

In fact, mature coping mechanisms generate *more* vitality for coping, showing an element of creativity and inspiration as well—marks of right-hemisphere originality. Mature coping mechanisms not only help people deal with difficult situations, but they actually give us more energy and stamina to do so. For instance, while the woman mentioned above was feeling fatigue and a low level of control related to her father's condition, she lifted her spirits and felt empowered by imagining something altruistic that she could do later of her own free will. In contrast, trying to cope by insisting that reality should change or by taking frustrations out on other people comes at a high cost.

I also would add *perspective* and *finding meaning or purpose* to George E. Vaillant's list of higher-end coping mechanisms. These ways of looking at life go a long way toward calming a person and enabling them to face hardship with more equanimity and peace. These mindsets widen our viewpoint from emotional reactivity to a broader perspective that soothes and uplifts us, helping us to feel less powerless in immediate circumstances.

Why More Mature Coping Mechanisms Matter

More mature coping isn't just a way of making yourself feel better in the moment. George E. Vaillant's review of long-term, longitudinal adult development studies found that better mental and physical health were associated with more mature coping mechanisms, while more symptomatic people showed less mature coping mechanisms (Vaillant, G. E., 1993).

The reason for this can be understood by recognizing that poorly managed stress places excessive demands on the body, causing fatigue and lowering vitality. When a person uses immature defense mechanisms, they end up *increasing* their stress and losing more energy. How a person grapples with stress will affect not only their mood, but their actual body functioning (Sapolsky, 1994/1998; van der Kolk, 2014). Our level of coping maturity determines how much energy we have to meet the challenge.

Chapter Wrap-Up

Helping ACEIPs regain self-awareness and improved vitality starts with teaching them to pay close attention to their own thoughts and feelings, while examining the self-stories and fate-narratives they may have pieced together from their early family roles. By focusing on your client's inner psychological world, you connect them to the source of their vitality and individuality. Your client gains strength from connecting with and expressing their feelings, while resolving the inhibiting reactions and beliefs that dampen their spontaneity, individuality, and unique interests. Vitality also depends on improved boundaries and working through healing fantasies, grief, and resentments. "Boring" sessions are signs of passive ACEIP adaptations and overly polite therapists, and should be deliberately steered into deeper explorations, with the therapist leading the way. Therapy progress shows in your client's improved access to their inner world, a stronger sense of self, reduced reactivity, more metaphorical and free associational communications, and more mature coping mechanisms. Having more mature coping mechanisms means you generate more energy by dealing with life's challenges realistically and on your own terms, using *both* left-brain rationality and right-brain insight and creativity.

Keep in Mind

- People make sense of their lives through stories, including fate-narratives. When you make these explicit, your client can begin to choose the self-stories they intend to live by.

- Progress shouldn't just be measured by decreases in symptoms or problems, but also by increased vitality and energy.

- Self-awareness has to be robust before a person can feel healthily entitled to their own personhood, boundaries, and individuality.

- People who get back in touch with themselves begin to speak in engaged and vivid ways that have a fresh metaphorical and freely associating style.

Chapter 7

The Primacy of Feelings

If therapy were a culture, emotions would be its language. At the beginning of a therapy relationship, we explain to our clients that feelings are messages from the true self, and their way back to knowing themselves. You know they've gotten it when they tear up and say something like: "There must be something here. I can feel myself getting emotional."

To me, the "tells" of emotional arousal are like road signs directing us toward what matters. I may direct clients back to a point where I noticed some emotion—a significant look, a hitch in their voice, or tears in their eyes—"Right there, when you said that, what were you feeling?" I look at these signs as indicators that the right-brain hemisphere has slipped some emotional truth through the left-brain's screen of words, inviting us to get real. I always try to say yes to that invitation.

Feelings are an embodied aspect of our experience that can only respond honestly. The true self knows what it knows and can't be talked out of its feelings by words and concepts.

So when an ACEIP client is moved to the point of emotion in a session, it's a very big deal. Even if you're in the middle of your intake interview, their feelings let you know that therapy has started. They're sensing adequate safety (Porges & Porges, 2023) and showing a bit of hope and trust in you and this new venture. Take advantage of this openness you have helped create with your therapeutic presence and stick with their feelings. You can always gather more data later.

Your job in receiving their feelings is to let them know you get it and want to know more. Sitting attentively, showing connection and interest on your face, making little sounds of interest and understanding—all these signs show them that they are on the right track and that you are genuinely interested. As you are listening, allow yourself to be curious. When there's an opportunity, ask them to tell you a little more about a feeling you thought you heard, or ask them to explain why something affected them as deeply as it clearly did. If you suspect other feelings that aren't spoken, inquire about them, but in an open-ended way that is not suggesting what they should've felt or not.

Feelings Might Be Unknown

ACEIPs may lack confidence in their feelings in part because they may not know exactly what to call them, having received little help from their EI parents in identifying and expressing emotions. Some feelings may not fit the ACEIP's familiar, conscious definition of themselves. Sometimes when these real feelings take over, ACEIPs don't understand how they can be feeling something so different from who they think they are or should be. They may even say, "That's not *me!*" But once your client's feelings start speaking up, they may have to enlarge their ideas about themselves as they get closer to their true self.

Self-knowledge develops quickly when a person starts listening to how they feel, and self-knowledge is the main ingredient for self-confidence. That's why it's important for therapists and their ACEIP clients to privilege emotion (Fosha, 2004; Johnson, S. M., 2019) in every encounter. ACEIPs have been deprived of help in dealing with their feelings, making it all the more important to provide it in therapy.

Because ACEIPs grew up around parents who acted nervous or defensive around real feelings and intimate conversations, they may see strong feelings as taboo, and even dangerous to relationship stability. Because their feelings often provoked anxious tension or even anger in their EI parents, many ACEIPs grew up feeling they were doing something wrong by being emotional.

They also have had the experience in the past of feeling *worse* after giving in to their feelings. They may have felt worse because showing their feelings to an emotionally unnurturing parent made them feel lonelier than they did before. The EI parent may have made them feel bad about "losing control," being "dramatic," "overreacting," or being "too sensitive." They may have limited experience with how sharing your true feelings with an empathic person makes you feel heard and relieved, and thus better. Your client can finally have this experience of emotional safety and acceptance as you resonate with them, show empathy, and accept their feelings as true.

This doesn't mean that as a therapist you have to force it or pretend to feel more than you do. All any client is really looking for is a sense that their therapist is reliably interested and compassionate toward them and their feelings. You may naturally be more reserved or more expressive: you can respond in whatever way is most authentic and comfortable, as long as you somehow communicate that you are taking your client seriously and that their feelings matter.

Supporting Your Client's Emotional Sensitivity

Growing up with EI parents can create a pattern of shame and discomfort around expressing feelings. It's likely that your client's EI parent didn't see your client's emotions as a strength or something to celebrate. That job might fall to you as their therapist.

When parents are afraid of emotional intimacy, children can grow up feeling they're too much for other people. They feel bad for breaking down at times, and they worry that their true feelings seem strange to others. They have no sense of their emotions as desirable indicators of their perceptiveness, sensitivity, or intuitions. That's why—when you get a chance—it's good to clearly acknowledge (and even celebrate) when your ACEIP client is being open and emotionally honest with you.

Since your ACEIP client has probably not had anyone wanting to hear *more* about their feelings when they were growing up, you in your therapist role are rectifying that. You also are in a position to bring attention to their emotional gifts and positive self-qualities whenever these stand out to you. It's very nurturing and strengthening to ACEIPs when someone recognizes their kindness, empathy, compassion, or sensitivity as highly desirable attributes that are crucial for relationships and parenting. When you hear your client has done something decent, caring, fair, or collaborative, comment on that as well. You thereby help them incorporate these positive human characteristics into their explicit, conscious self-concept.

The Gifted Client

Very intelligent or gifted clients even have what is called *over-excitability* or *super-sensibility*: a capacity for heightened emotion, sensitivity, and perceptiveness described by psychiatrist and giftedness researcher Kazimierz Dabrowski (1964/2016; Daniels & Piechowski, 2009). For a gifted individual, the low empathy and insensitivity of EI parents can be especially hurtful. Their sensitivity is generally a psychological burden for them, so it is especially meaningful to them that someone has noticed their deep feelings and strong sense of altruism. If you think a client is highly intelligent or gifted, I suggest reading in the gifted literature on the unique psychological challenges such people face (Daniels & Piechowski, 2009; Mendaglio, 2008; Ruf, 2023). If you do so, you may be one of the few people they have come across who truly gets them.

EIPs Classify Feelings as "Right" or "Wrong"

Protecting themselves with left-brained certainties, EIPs often categorize everything rigidly, as good or bad, right or wrong. Unless their children keep to the level of feelings they can tolerate, they can make their children feel ashamed or guilty. They might punish a child's anger or expect their sadness to clear up immediately so the parent can move on. In such a family climate, there's no way for a child to explore the reasons for their feelings or to express them without feeling bad for having them. This particularly is true of anger, which the EIP's child is expected to suppress, potentially leading to lifetime feelings of powerlessness and resentment.

One ACEIP summarized her emotional experience growing up by saying that, to her parents, "My feelings made no sense; my problems were meaningless and had no purpose; I had to renounce my connection to my true self or be seen as selfish."

Sadly, most ACEIPs internalize their parents' attitudes toward their emotions. This makes it hard for them to allow themselves to feel things freely because they've learned that deep feelings mostly elicit criticism or disinterest. The disappointment of opening up to someone, showing your honest feelings, and then having the person react with disinterest, fact-finding, or evaluation feels unsafe to *anyone*. Giving your ACEIP client a welcoming place in therapy where feelings can emerge, and they can experience their inner emotional world without embarrassment, is a true gift.

The Therapist's Response to Feelings

To encourage your client to feel and explore their emotional experiences, it helps to explain to them why you think feelings are so important. You can tell them something like this:

> *I'm interested in all your feelings. They tell us what matters to you and how things affect you. Feelings don't care if something is small or big; they just care about the truth. So if we take feelings seriously, they will give us vital information about what we need.*

Your goal as therapist is the complete legitimization of your client's emotional experience (Miller, 1981). Nothing they feel is "small," "silly," or "unimportant." This welcoming attitude is crucial for therapy, since ACEIPs have been taught by EI parents to discount their emotional lives. It can take quite a while for a client to get comfortable enough to just sit with a feeling and see what's there.

As therapist, you may be the first person who has shown interest in translating your ACEIP client's feelings into words. EI parents often act as if their children's feelings are meaningless artifacts, unnecessary and better off suppressed. More emotionally aware parents naturally use a feeling-informed vocabulary with their children, making it easy for them to learn and use the names for emotions. As psychologist and neuroscientist Lisa Barrett (2017) explains, children aren't born recognizing various emotions. Initially, they only have body sensations that must be understood and named by the older people around them. This means that the parent has to have enough empathy and self-reflection to accurately imagine the emotional state of the child and give it a name.

Since EI parents lack these processing skills, their children don't get this assistance, and end up often feeling confused and overwhelmed by their emotions, with no healthy way to integrate them into their personalities. Instead, they may strive for surface emotional control while struggling with undercurrents of raw, unprocessed emotion. In such a scenario, it's easy to see why they would be reluctant to go deeply into their feelings: they're not only afraid of what they'll find, they're afraid that if their deeper emotional life comes out, it will disrupt their hard-won emotional control.

A version of this fear occurs when people stop themselves from crying because they're afraid that if they start, they'll never stop. They learn this from emotionally phobic (McCullough et al., 2003) parents who fear emotion as a powerful alien force that will take you over if you're not careful. If a client habitually bottles up their emotion in a session, you can say something like this:

> *I know to you these feelings seem strong and kind of scary. But you know, human beings are designed to experience all kinds of emotions, and really deep ones too. We don't start crying and never stop; that would be impossible. I know it can feel that way, but feelings come in waves. They peak and fall off [using cresting-wave hand gesture] as soon as we let them out. I think somebody probably was uncomfortable with your emotions, and made you feel that way too. Do you think that's possible?*

Facilitating Emotional Expression and Exploration

If a person is having a hard time putting their feelings into words, you might get them started by offering guesses about how something made them feel. You can rely on your empathy and mentalization abilities (Fonagy et al., 2002) to imagine the kind of reaction they're probably experiencing, long before they are able to put their feelings into words. Other clients are so clear about their feelings that all you have to do is keep up. But you can still help them explore and clarify their feelings, helping them to round out their sense of self, understand their needs, and integrate their emotional life into their overall personality.

If a client really struggles with putting their feelings into words, don't be discouraged. Let them know you get it *without words*. Accelerated Experiential Dynamic Psychotherapy (AEDP) founder Diana Fosha (2000) has encouraged therapists to tell clients they don't have to know how to express feelings because they are so eloquent with just their face and eyes. This takes the burden to name everything off the client, truly a relief when feelings are subtle or complex. Parents do this all the time with their children. The adequately sensitive parent registers the child's face and body expressions, recognizes the associated feelings through their mirror neurons (Rizolatti, 2005; Rizolatti & Craighero, 2004), and makes a very good guess of what the child is probably feeling.

Use a kind, unobtrusive style and start where the client is, even if their emotional expression isn't very verbal yet. If a client is sitting silently, fiddling with a tissue with tears in their eyes, you could ask them to help you understand what their hands and tears would say if they could. Since so many people just aren't comfortable talking about their feelings, they might reply with "I don't know" when asked. Perhaps they're afraid to say the wrong thing. You can reply: "Well, yes, of course you don't *know*. But...if you *did* know, what do you think it would be?"

If you sense that the person wants to open up their about feelings but isn't sure what's normal in this therapy situation, try *proxy speech* (Johnson, S. M., 2019). In this method, the therapist starts talking as if they were the voice of the client's inner experience, putting their feelings into the everyday language that many people might use to express the same thing. For instance, the therapist might say out loud what they imagine the client might be feeling or thinking in the situation they're describing, such as "And you're there wanting to say to them, like, *did you ever think about how that affects me?*"). You're showing a willingness to guess your client's feelings or thoughts under those conditions—letting them know that you're trying to get it. You're also modeling a willingness to be wrong, and to be corrected by them. If you miss the mark, ask them to correct and refine your statement ("*Oh good, I want to be accurate here. What* did *go through your mind?*"). Sometimes giving them something to work with, something to correct, makes it much easier for your client to get started.

Building Emotional Granularity

As a therapist, you'll be trying to match your client's feelings with the right word, not just a ballpark "mad, sad, glad" designation. This is emotional *granularity* (Barrett, 2017), which develops as a person refines the distinctions among their feelings. For instance, the general feeling of anger could be further honed into terms like frustrated, irritated, annoyed, agitated, aggravated, angry, incensed, infuriated, or enraged. Sadness could be expressed as touched, moved, sorry, melancholy, blue, down, sorrowful, grief-stricken, or anguished. It's all about understanding our inner experiences, identifying what feelings are trying to tell us about how situations are impacting us. Emotions are the best indicators of well-being or threat that we have. They certainly are quicker than left-brain analysis, and they tell us what we need to know to take care of ourselves.

In addition to regular, discrete emotions, you can also help clients describe those more ephemeral *vitality affects* (Stern, 1985) that we learned about in chapter 6: dynamic, *fluid* patterns of experiences such as sensing an uplift, a burst of creative inspiration, a downshift in mood, the flooding of exuberance, the drain of devitalization, kinetic joy, surging mood changes, or any other feeling-state that sends a wave of affect or sensation through us as we move through time.

the best thing *for the client* at that moment. In my practice, I don't touch my clients because I don't see that as the nature of our work together. My job is to help them to explore and communicate their feelings, while I do my best to support and understand. I respond as calmly and genuinely as I can, with my words, eyes, facial expressions, and body language. Using physical touch in therapy has many possible implications, some of which you may never have intended. In my opinion, there's such an interpersonal power imbalance inherent in the therapist-client relationship that touch can never be perceived as a neutral event. If you engage in touch once, will something be perceived as being amiss if you don't the next time? Or will you as therapist possibly worry whether you should touch the client again this time, once it's on the table? Personally, I prefer to keep the lines straight and put my energy into expressing my empathy in other ways.

You may sincerely believe a situation is exceptional and that some sort of caring touch is the best response. Perhaps a client has fallen into real despair over a situation and is tuning everything out but their own anguish, and you don't feel you're reaching them any other way. But just be aware that even aside from ethical issues it may cause, physical touch that is not part of your original agreement with your client is a wild card. Of course you would process it with them afterwards; still, it's so unusual to be touched by your therapist that it may well not be as comforting as you intend it to be. You just don't know how the client is going to interpret your action.

It's always worth asking yourself if the urge to reach out to them may be coming from your own subconscious urge to calm them down. If it feels like it's not enough to just sit with them and convey empathy, ask yourself if you might be overidentifying with or amplifying the client's pain or taking responsibility for making them feel better. Maybe they don't need to feel better so much as they need to learn that they are capable of withstanding their emotional experiences once they feel accepted and understood.

Even the seemingly innocuous offer of a tissue may suggest you're getting uncomfortable, or finding their tears "messy" and in need of a clean-up. Wait for the client to show some desire for a tissue (looking around, acting like *they* need one, etc.) before offering it, or indicating where the box is. Immediately offering a mop-up is less effective than showing with your eyes or posture or any of a hundred ways that you're with them and care—that you're comfortable with crying.

Additionally, offering tissues is a pro forma social response, something people do to be polite. It's kind, but it's appropriate to a *social* situation, not necessarily to a therapeutic one. Your job is to convey that they should feel free to let their feelings out, even if it means a runny nose. You don't want them worrying whether the therapist is going to jump in with a tissue or a reaching hand the moment they start to feel their feelings at last. The values and goals of psychotherapy are completely different from those of a social encounter.

If a client wonders why you are *not* showing physical support when they're upset, simply explain why you don't, including any of the reasons noted above. Sometimes people don't know what to expect, and you have to explain the unique norms of the therapy relationship, and how it is for their ultimate benefit. In the unlikely event that a client takes offense or accuses you of being cold or unfeeling because you haven't offered a shoulder or a handhold, you can validate their feelings but assure them that therapy is about learning to explore and handle feelings together, not necessarily making them feel better right away. (If you feel pressured or shamed by the client to show more closeness than you're comfortable with, consider that they may be using projective identification to unconsciously demonstrate how it felt to them to be coerced out of their boundaries by the EIPs in their life.)

Whatever the reason, it helps to explain the therapeutic rationale and boundary observance behind your decisions. But you're not accountable for making them happy about it. You are responsible for taking care of yourself and (ultimately) your client by sticking to a way of therapy that you're comfortable with and that doesn't exhaust you or threaten your own boundaries.

Challenging Their Emotional Overidentification

Why is your ACEIP client so prone to overidentify with the suffering of others? (And if you are an ACEIP yourself, consider that you might be at risk for the same overidentification with your client's feelings.) Overidentification can be a combination of boundary problems and psychological enmeshment with the other person, both of which are potential pitfalls when a person has had an EI parent. Such clients learn that their existence should revolve around helping their parent maintain emotional stability and self-esteem. For many ACEIPs, this blurring of boundaries and feeling responsible for the psychological well-being of another person just feels normal.

Overidentification is very different from offering support and empathy to a loved one. Even if you love someone very much and want to help them any way you can, the sufficiently emotionally mature person doesn't lose their sense of self in the process. They're still aware of their own feelings and reactions and retain a sense of themselves as a separate person.

Overidentification based on psychological enmeshment with another person has a particular vibe. There is a sense that your client has dived headfirst into the other person's problem, making them nearly as distressed as the other person. They go beyond empathy, working themselves up to feel the level of suffering they imagine the other person is going through, as if true love and loyalty meant matching their level of distress. (It is likely that this overboard empathy is what an EI parent expected.)

Later in life, overidentification shows up when a person claims to know exactly what someone is going through. They seem to worry and suffer as much as, if not more than, the other person. Many times, I've had clients who were convinced they were feeling the exact feelings of the other person. Whenever I hear that, I take it as my therapist's job to question this assumption, as I don't think it's a healthy or even reality-based approach to relationships. I don't concur with the idea that closeness means you *actually* feel the same thing as the other person.

I remind such clients that we can surmise someone's feelings—and sometimes very accurately—but we can't crawl inside their skin to feel what they feel. I remind them that everyone is a separate person and that even on our best days, we still can only guess what goes on in other people. Intimate communication is how we get that information: we must *ask* another person how they're feeling, what a situation means to them, and so on. I encourage clients to start with the respectful assumption that none of us are psychic when it comes to other people's feelings, and that interest, curiosity, and empathy develop relationships more deeply than assuming you already know what they're feeling.

Overimagining EIPs' Pain

Ironically, what an ACEIP imagines their EIP is going through is likely to be worse than what the person is actually experiencing. The ACEIP imagines what they themselves—with all their sensitivity—would feel and then probably end up feeling worse than the EIP does. EIPs' actual distress is probably less acute because their defense mechanisms protect them from getting too upset. In fact, if you listen carefully to what EIPs are most upset about, you'll mostly hear themes of anger, betrayal, victimization, or self-pity crowding out more acute feelings of sadness, grief, regret, or guilt. They may seem very emotional, but many times you'll note a deep complaint wedged in there somewhere, with the pointed implication that someone should do something about it.

This is not to minimize the fact that many EIPs have had trauma in their life, with plenty of reasons to be upset. But they avoid deeper feelings even when they're displaying big reactions. They just don't take things to heart in the same way that the internalizer ACEIP imagines because they're not internal processers.

As a therapist, you can propose the radical idea that your client may be suffering for their EIP more than the EIP is suffering for themselves, and that perhaps it's unnecessary to immerse themselves in the other person's pain to this degree. This may be confusing to the ACEIP because they have been taught that self-suffering is the best way to show you really care about someone. They learned this from EIPs who subconsciously transfer their pain to others, to get them to feel what they can't themselves. That's the whole function of projective identification: *join me and feel what I can't afford to be conscious of.* Remember, EIPs only feel loved when someone "proves" it by self-sacrificing for them.

Your client needs to know it's okay to feel empathy for the other person, but without loaning out their own heart as an amplifier for the other person's unprocessed pain. It is often a revelation to the ACEIP to think that just a normal amount of empathy and concern still counts as caring. They think showing love means suffering alongside them, because EIPs typically don't feel better until someone else is feeling worse.

Try saying to your client: *I know you love them. I know you're concerned about them. But do you really have to turn yourself inside out to prove that to them? Is it necessary to get torn up over what you're imagining they're going through? What would happen if you just felt empathy and concern and stopped there?*

Overidentification as Secret Self-Nurturing

ACEIPs who have been unnurtured emotionally can derive secret, subconscious pleasure and self-nurturing from feeling great concern over the emotional needs of others. This is the alchemy of the *sublimation* defense: transforming a past of painful deprivation into the present-day pursuit of altruism and generosity. Rather than realizing what we have missed in our own lives, our high imaginative capacity can prompt us to give others what we needed ourselves. We thus unconsciously get our needs met indirectly through identifying with someone else's experience of being given to. However, sometimes sublimation works so well that we ourselves are actually transformed—the satisfaction of wanting to help becomes its own reward.

Helping ACEIPs Recognize and Process Their Feelings

Our emotions arise from our limbic brain structures, which are largely processed by the right hemisphere for an immediate gut feel of contextual danger or safety, then on to the left hemisphere for more analysis, as each hemisphere contributes its take on meaning and needed actions. Our analytic and sequential left brain names the feeling, looks for immediate linear cause and effect of the emotion, and puts our experience into words so it can be consciously thought about or relayed to others. In a well-integrated mind, like a good team player, the left brain respectfully defers to our right hemisphere for processing context, broader meanings, and a huge associational array of other considerations, perhaps ultimately leading to wider insights or profound self-realizations. A feeling is fully processed when it involves all these aspects of the brain (Taylor, J. B., 2021; Schore, 2009). EIPs tend to do poorly at brain integrating and processing, either getting stuck in emotional upheaval or keeping a death-grip on left-brained certainty and judgment while denying right-brained contextual awareness.

Integrated emotional processing translates our experiences into consciousness in a way that provides a sense of self and meaning in life. The more we feel and identify our feelings—linking their present meanings to our memories—the more emotional depth and wisdom we have, both for ourselves and other people. Under good-enough conditions, our emotional processing function becomes increasingly integrated within our brain as we grow up, and some lucky people even have parents who are empathic and interested enough to teach them how to process their experiences in this way.

But self-preoccupied EI parents aren't good at attending to their child's emotional experiences in the first place, so they certainly are not taking the time to empathize with the child's feelings and help them put names on those feelings. Unknowingly, they leave their children to be swamped by feelings, without guiding them in how to grow from the experience nor expanding their self-awareness and self-knowledge.

Such a child is left to wrestle with emotional pain or to feel in a jumble, with no help making sense of all these sensations coursing through their body. Without cognitive structure to help in identifying and naming feelings in all their variations (i.e., bringing in the talents of the orderly left brain), the child's mind is not strengthened by an awareness of emotion, but instead feels threatened by it. In such a scenario, they learn that feeling strong emotion only leads to distress and even helplessness. Without support in intellectually mastering and integrating their emotions, the child might feel they are limited to restrictive choices for how to deal with their feelings: for example, keeping distance from their feelings, suppressing them from conscious thought, dissociating from the experience, or finding other ways to ignore emotions that have no path to integration and mastery within the child's personality.

Years later, you the therapist will notice your client's tragic compartmentalization of what should have developed into a vibrant, complexly integrated personality structure and self-story. You now encounter your ACEIP client still struggling with emotion, holding at bay many of their feelings, and out of touch with vital right-brain tools such as imagery, metaphor, imagination, self-awareness, and intuition. Often they have abandoned their unprocessed emotions, sensations, and arousals and fled into the wordy left brain in an attempt to become a respectable, grown-up person. They still have their emotional sensitivity, of course, but without a good way to conceptualize and appreciate it, they mistrust it in themselves.

Therapists who are ACEIPs themselves may also need to do their own therapy work around getting acquainted and comfortable with their own unexamined childhood feelings. On the positive side, this deep reservoir of intense, unprocessed childhood emotion can provide the raw material for a special kind of empathy for your clients, plus it helps you understand how passionate feelings can sweep over a person, despite their best intentions. Your own unresolved issues with emotion can make you a more humane and compassionate therapist, as long as you have addressed them consciously and learned from the experience.

Make Friends with Their Left Brain First

Start with topics your client experiences as safe. If someone has learned to live comfortably and safely in a snug hovel, they might not appreciate your well-meaning attempts to uproot them and move them to a large and airy mansion. They might feel quite exposed and lost, as if ejected from their container. If a very rational ACEIP client has found safety and self-esteem living in their verbal and orderly left-brain hemisphere, you can't expect them to immediately trust you and throw open the door to their feelings and urges. Worse, they just don't understand what you're talking about.

Consequently, when you ask them how they *feel*, they're likely to tell you what they *think*. They have no idea how to consult themselves at an emotional level. It's common in left-brain-biased, techno-industrial societies that many very successful people don't exactly know what you're getting at when you ask them how they feel about something. They think you're asking for their opinion or evaluation of the subject.

Now, this is an interesting misunderstanding, and you can make it interesting to them too. You can neutrally point out to them that you asked about a feeling, and they gave you a thought. This may be repeated a few times while they claim they really have no feelings at the moment. That, you can be sure, is *not* the problem. We're all having feelings all the time. The problem is that your client has trained themselves not to be in touch with the sensations of emotions in the presence of an authority figure, possibly because it could make their feelings of loneliness and vulnerability worse. They don't yet believe that you are truly on their side. They think you're looking for them to be well-behaved and smart, like their parents did, and to not bother you too much with inexplicably messy and ambivalent feelings.

So you can partner with their left-brain skills by explaining how necessary feelings are to our sense of self, our confidence, and our ability to know what we want in life. You can tell them how important it is to get in touch with their feelings, and that you will help them with that because it's going to open their life up. You inform them that all human beings are very emotional and sensitive, and that feelings-awareness (or emotional intelligence, as Daniel Goleman [1995] described it) is crucial for satisfying relationships and a meaningful life.

After your promotion of emotional awareness, you might wonder with them if they had some early experiences that convinced them otherwise? How were feelings handled in their family? What did they do—and what did other people do—when they got upset? What feelings were frowned upon? What kinds of emotions were permitted at home?

By doing this kind of emotional history-taking, you are helping your client to realize how their feelings were not supported—or even how they were made to feel bad about having them. This emerging narrative of their emotional past will begin to pull them back into their own life story, through left-brain time sequencing, but also through their right hemisphere's integrative ability to find meaningful context for understanding themselves.

They return to being a main character in their own story. Through gaining a sense of what happened to their trust in their feelings, they begin to understand and care about the person they've become in a newly protective way.

How Growth Feelings Show Up

In AEDP, Diana Fosha (2000, 2009) has researched the kinds of feelings in psychotherapy that are associated with transformational experiences, those moments when the person contacts new levels of self-realization and self-integrity. Such feelings are the evidence and energy of what Fosha calls *transformance,* a person's motivational drive toward "vitality, authenticity, adaptation, and coherence" and resultant growth (Fosha, 2009; p. 175). These transformational feelings are characterized by a "subjective sense of 'truth'" (p. 188) and contribute to attaining what she calls the *core state* of "calm, clarity, flow, and expansiveness" (Fosha, 2020) Many of my clients have also reported a distinct sense of spaciousness and wide-awake presence at these times.

When these core-state signs show up, halt any other therapy agenda and focus on noticing and amplifying what the client is experiencing. In chapter 9, we'll see how, when a client is helped to consciously experience, integrate, and appreciate this personal transformation, it becomes theirs to keep. The goal of these moments is to help the client keep their focus on their transformational affects, facilitating an upward spiral of making these feelings more and more conscious and real to the person.

But not all growth feels positive at first. Remember that sometimes when people are undergoing major changes in psychotherapy, they experience the psychological discombobulation of *positive disintegration* (Dabrowski, 1964/2016). When a person is changing and growing psychologically, they often feel preoccupied, off-kilter, or not quite right. Growth loosens up our old foundations, so to speak, preparing us to accommodate and assimilate (Piaget, 1963) a new way of being in the world. This can feel disorienting until the person establishes a new level of intrapsychic organization within themselves. Children often go through these intervals of disequilibrium until they can reorganize themselves internally around their new level of learning and development (Ilg et al., 1981).

Interestingly, internalizer ACEIPs—who love to process and learn—keep on growing psychologically as they age, with the result that they might often go through periods of disequilibrium or other "negative" feelings as they reorganize themselves at a new, more complex level. Conversely, an emotionally immature person might fear such growth disruptions as crises and react to them in regressive rather than maturing ways. Instead of trying to figure out what's happening or asking themselves questions about their life, as an internalizer might, an EIP is more likely to seek some immediate relief so they can get back to the status quo. The opportunity for psychological growth is lost, as the person desperately grabs at old certainties and distractions.

Other reasons internalizing ACEIPs turn toward growth opportunities are their greater tolerance for emotional complexity and their curiosity about and receptivity to their own inner experiences. Most ACEIPs like to understand their own psychological functioning: they enjoy thinking about things, talking to someone, or maybe journaling about them. They are much more likely than EIPs to sense significance in an uncomfortable feeling and want to understand its meaning.

As mentioned previously, more psychologically aware ACEIPs have more capacity to tolerate ambiguity, let things evolve, and not need to pin everything down. This means they're open to creative thought and have a mindset that seeks out connection and meaning, even in apparent disorder. It's the perfect attitude toward life to support and reinforce psychological development. When a person pursues meaning and growth, they are much more likely to rise out of a period of disequilibrium on an upward spiral, attaining new levels of confidence as their inner integration process catches up.

Being a therapist who's aware of normal growth upheavals in psychological development, whether for children or adults, helps you to reassure and guide your client when they feel out of sorts during a period of intense therapy or change. You can help them realize they need time to accommodate a high rate of growth before they feel more normal again. The affective difference between regression crises and growth crises is that in *growth*, the person feels a little preoccupied, distracted, or off balance, while in a psychological *regression*, there is more acute distress: their personality structures are not containing anxiety or fear very well, and there is an increase in psychological symptoms and acting out.

Feel-the-Feelings Techniques

When a person seems cut off from their feelings, they probably feel safer in the parts of their mind they consider rational or in control. You as therapist can work with that by explaining why feelings are so important (e.g., fuller and richer living, better relationships, stronger sense of self, better decision-making) and why you'll be asking about them. This helps to explicitly orient them to tune in to their emotional reactions. If your client has trouble getting in touch with their feelings, there are several things to try. Let's look at different techniques to help your client get to know their emotional life in more detail.

Point Out the Emotion-Body Connection

If a client seems at a loss in describing their feelings, or they use very simple, generic feeling-words without elaboration, ask them where they're feeling a reaction in their body as they talk about it. When they've pinpointed its location, ask them to describe it in words or with a metaphor.

You can also use a variation of Peter Levine's (1997) sensory, body-experiencing check-in by asking them more imaginative questions, such as "If that feeling had a color, what would it be? If you could touch that feeling, what would it feel like? If that feeling had a temperature, what would it be? If the feeling had a smell, what would it be like?" and so on. Sometimes this exercise leads people deeper into associations and experience, getting to know their feelings in a more embodied way. Other times, it might seem like more trouble than it's worth for its yield—nevertheless, it offers a shared right-brain immediacy of experience between you and your client that shows your sincere interest in wanting to know their inner experience.

Slow-Motion Expansion of Feelings

Most people are not accustomed to talking about their emotional reactions in detail, especially ACEIPs who have not yet learned how in therapy. They usually sum an experience up in a word or two, and move on. It's helpful to ask your client to zoom in on the moment where they started having an emotional reaction and report it as if it were happening in slow motion, so they can describe exactly what happened and how their reaction developed moment to moment.

When clients slow down and describe events and their feelings in the order they came into being, the real meaning of their reaction comes into focus. For instance, in a conversation with their EIP, maybe it turns out it wasn't exactly what the person said, but *how* they said it, with arched eyebrow or tight lips. To your client, this had a specific nonverbal meaning, based on painful past experiences. You wouldn't know this just listening to an overview of the encounter.

Feeling Feelings to Completion

This next approach is most useful when a client has been unable to process their feelings because either the EIP in their life didn't listen or shut them down, or because they just don't know how. Unfortunately, this only prolongs the painful emotion, because feelings don't disappear—they turn into buried, unfinished feelings (Truman, 1991/2003).

In the session, explain to your client that it's important to get to the bottom of their feeling. Using Diana Fosha's (2000, 2020) recommended warm and engaging style, you will keep them focused on what they're feeling: *"Just stick with it, let's see what's underneath that feeling... Good! And what else?... Yes, and what else?"* By focusing on their difficult feeling and gently returning to it as long as needed, you help them finally feel it through to completion (Gendlin, 1978; Fosha, 2000). (Note that feeling feelings to completion does *not* mean unleashing disorganizing levels of emotion to the point of causing flashbacks or retraumatizing your client.)

Here's an example of non-traumatic feeling to completion: your client might've been angrily obsessing over an argument, but when they kept processing to get to the heart of it, you find out the other person actually made them feel ashamed, like they were exposed as a bad person, a feeling that's been there all their life. By working through this underlying feeling, there will be a sense of completion, like you can't go any deeper than this. When the client discovers what the obsessive anger was really all about, they often have a quietly confessional tone, as though they're admitting something they didn't want to face. Now you both have the information and opportunity to go deeper into this feeling—what it's like, how it may have been running their life, what they think makes it true, and so forth.

If a person doesn't get to the bottom of the feeling in the session, or quickly moves away from the feeling no matter what you do, I recommend what I call "sitting in the dirty diaper." Encourage the client to practice staying in touch with the unpleasant feeling for a while, deliberately experiencing it without shutting it down immediately, like they want to. Tell them this will feel extremely noxious, like sitting in a dirty diaper, but it is an effective way to get to know their emotions and needs at a deeper level.

You can use this technique in your own life, especially if there is a situation that you're obsessing over. By deliberately dropping down into the feeling and staying there, perhaps journaling your thoughts as you sit there, you can feel it to completion instead of spinning in your thoughts on the surface.

Panic, Rage, and Overwhelming Emotion

Rage and panic are deeply physical feelings. All emotions start in the body, but these two feelings have a unique urgency toward physical expression. They are based in the fight-or-flight sympathetic autonomic nervous system response, creating almost irresistible urges to take action.

Panic: A Survival Reflex

In many modern cultures that value left-brain logic above all, panic gets a bad reputation as losing control and showing weakness. But in all animals, panic is a survival reflex, forcing us to act, to get away at all costs. The escape reflexes of panic are a last-ditch effort to do whatever we can to save ourselves. However, if a threatening situation occurs that demands desperate escape, but the person either believes escape is impossible or they're too terrified to move, that physical arousal can get stuck in the body. EI parents can trigger chronic unresolved panic in their children because they often create emotionally contradictory situations in which a child feels damned if they do and damned if they don't.

In his book on trauma, *Waking the Tiger* (1997), Peter Levine discusses how trauma can get stuck in the body when a person holds the pent-up, unexpressed energy of fear and need to escape. He shares an exercise of helping a client imagine themselves back in the terrifying or overwhelming situation, encouraging them to *feel* what their body wants to *do* at that moment, and then to *express* it in some kind of physical movement. In this way, the person not only has an opportunity to feel the feeling to completion but to complete the action too. For instance, by emotionally imagining, pantomiming, or acting out uncompleted survival reactions such as running away as fast as they can, vehemently pushing someone away, or speaking out against what's happening in order to stop the situation, the original natural self-defending response gets an outlet. Of course, as a therapist, you must have experience dealing with trauma and know your client's ability to retain some capacity for self-observation here, so you don't run the risk of re-traumatizing them.

The idea with Levine's technique is to have the client stay grounded with you in the session while imagining the traumatic situation vividly, feeling it in their body, and then sensing what the body is telling them to do. Instead of immersing in it like an uncontrolled flashback, you're encouraging the client to make movements and gestures while putting it into words—describing their fantasy of what they wish they could've done in the past situation. They can move the muscle groups involved in a kind of pantomime of their feelings. The goal is that they go beneath the stuck feelings to the underlying, unexpressed bodily impulses in a way that feels real, but safe. Having these primitive and life-saving impulses accepted and encouraged by one's therapist allows the person to feel the healthy impulses behind their panic and to move past feeling utterly helpless and frozen.

Rage: A Reaction to Threat

Rage is another natural reaction to threats to our safety and survival. It, too, creates powerful physical urges, usually to overcome or destroy whatever has tried to control or threaten us. ACEIP clients often feel terribly guilty or ashamed of experiencing rage if they feel that way toward EIPs they love or are attached to. Rage can build when the child is excessively controlled and judged by the parent, or when boundary violations by EI parents and a refusal to respect the ACEIP's individuality can create an infuriating atmosphere of unfairness. Nevertheless, they've been taught by EI parents that their anger is unwarranted, extreme, and requires repression. The child is made to feel that *they* have overreacted and there is something wrong with them for having such an angry response.

It is often a big part of therapy work with ACEIPs to go back and investigate the sources of rage. Many times, the ACEIP has disowned the feeling and filled it in with symptoms of anxiety or depression instead. For example, the ACEIP might have swallowed their rage when the parent used them as a confidant, burdening them with things they didn't want to hear. Or maybe the parent violated their personal boundaries or autonomy, using them as an object for their needs, creating what are often called "icky" or "yucky" feelings. Your job is to grasp how it may have made them feel when their parent did these rage-provoking things—infuriating and exasperating them but then forbidding them to express it.

Rage makes us want to scream, hit something, or destroy something. If unacknowledged and bottled up, rage can show up as confusion, pressure-cooker tension, and a powerful urge to take action. But once clients identify rage, you can help them find safe ways to express it, so that the feeling has a natural action outlet to accompany whatever insights you may discover.

For instance, one client described to me how he had dealt with overwhelming unfair pressure at work by going out to his car and screaming his frustrations. Later, he could address the work situation with constructive plans, but for that moment, he was emotionally stuck, and his rage craved an outlet. Another client discovered that when she was on her last nerve parenting little children all day, going in the bathroom and angrily biting or squeezing a towel helped her not take it out on the kids. Any similar action is preferable to acting out rage with people in ways that might be potentially destructive to all involved. Feeling less rage is a *future* goal; but sometimes something physical has to be done *now* with the feelings that have come up. Along with physical expression, the experience needs to be talked about and integrated into the client's self-understanding and emotional awareness. Clients can own and feel the legitimacy of their rage feelings while they learn to understand and channel them into more constructive insight and action.

Overwhelming Emotions

In therapy, there are times when we want to explore emotional experiences, such as those discussed above, but there can be times when a person is in danger of reliving trauma or a flashback from PTSD (post-traumatic stress disorder). Flashbacks are not just feelings of panic and rage, but actual retraumatization by re-experiencing the trauma as if it were happening again now. In order to know what to do in such moments, you have to have training in managing and dealing with trauma, which is beyond the scope of this book. But if you get caught unaware in an unexpected onslaught of client emotion, I can suggest a handful of approaches that you might use if you're trying to help a client regroup from an emotional overload. The following methods are not intended to treat trauma directly, but they can help you teach them how to regulate overwhelming emotion when they're not ready for it or are feeling panicky.

Ask the Part to Step Back

Suggest to your client that there is a part of their personality coming forward that is carrying a lot of emotion, but maybe they're not ready to take it on right now. Internal Family Systems (IFS) therapy (Schwartz, 1995), a modality we'll talk about more in the next chapter, suggests asking the client to imagine requesting that this emotional part of the personality please take a step back. You could say to your client:

Tell that part that you are interested and do want to know what it's feeling, but that we need to do it in a way that isn't too overwhelming. Ask the part if it's willing to move back and give you a chance to regroup. Be sure to thank it as you do so, since it's only trying to help. We're not going to abandon it; we just need some time and space to get used to what it needs to tell us.

Use Emotional Distancing Techniques

This could be followed by other self-protective IFS methods, such as familiarizing oneself with the part by imagining looking at it in a room with a two-way mirror or seeing it at a distance from you—just observing it at first. Without the immediate threat of feeling overwhelmed by all the suppressed emotion bursting out, your client may be able to generate much more empathy and understanding of those emotionally injured parts of themselves.

You could help them find other ways of expressing these feelings, through drawings, expressive movements or dance, looking at childhood photographs, or journaling in the part's voice, whatever they're comfortable with. These sublimations of raw emotion express feelings in ways that modulate them at the same time. By putting these initially overwhelming feelings into art or creative expression, they begin to be transformed by the intrapsychic processes that integrate activities in the thinking, artistic, and feeling parts of the brain.

Ground Them in the Present Moment

You can orient clients back to the present moment by guiding them, through mindfulness (Siegel, D. J., 2010a; Siegel, R. D., 2010) to the feel of the chair they're sitting on, their feet on the floor, their breath going in and out, the sounds around them. This reconnection with the present sensory moment helps people regain their footing, emotionally speaking, and feel more in control.

Remind Them: "It's just a feeling"

If your client isn't able to stop the slide into overwhelming affect, you may have to just sit with them through it, letting them know that you're right there with them, reassuring them they're doing a good job, and that these are just the feelings that they have never been allowed to express. You could say something like:

[Name], *you seem like you're feeling* [name feeling]. *Do you think that's what it is right now?* [Get confirmation or correction of the emotion.] *What a difficult feeling that is—it's almost too much to face, isn't it? But this is just a feeling. That's all it is. You're having the feeling; it's not having you. The feeling is inside you; you are not inside it. This feeling is really strong, but this feeling is not the end of the world; it just feels like it... You haven't lost touch with everything familiar in your life, I'm right here with you. I think this was from a long time ago. I think it's showing you that this is how bad it was... It was too big for you then... But you can feel it now... We can feel it together... Good for you.*

As you are helping them complete their emotional processing and you are understanding them accurately, you're helping them see the feelings as an *experience* that can be dealt with instead of something overwhelming that feels like the end of the *world*. (This can be helpful only if you don't skip the first step of empathizing with how awful it legitimately feels to your client.)

Define the Feeling

Try to identify the main tone of the feeling that is washing over them; it might be shame, guilt, regret, or something else. Putting words on the feeling shrinks the overwhelm back to the status of a feeling by naming it and expressing empathy with how distressing it is. This is what a good parent might do with a very upset child: first honoring their feelings, then reminding them that you and they will be together through this. If you think the feeling is from your client's long ago past, you can define the feeling as something that they've never been able to process, but now they can. This promotes a sense of efficacy, activating the left brain and corralling the feelings into a delineated space within the client's sequential life-narrative.

Chapter Wrap-Up

Feelings are primary in psychotherapy with ACEIPs. Many of their emotional experiences have been shut down by the EIPs in their lives and need to be reanimated in their therapy. By establishing emotional resonance, right brain to right brain, the therapist creates a bridge back to the client's sense of self and emotional validity. Extremely influential implicit memories can be made conscious by following the trail of feelings back to the client's early implicit learnings about the self and the world. Growth upheavals need to be differentiated from more regressive or symptomatic feelings. Feeling feelings to completion helps the client understand and integrate the original message of the emotion. When needed, there are methods to help them regain emotional control, so as not to feel retraumatized. By focusing on feeling their feelings, clients discover the original meaning of their emotional experiences and their legitimate place in their lives.

Parts work is good for therapists too. If you as therapist also do the work of identifying and understanding your own personality parts, you'll find your objectivity and compassion improving in sessions as well.

The Primary Importance of Empathy and Acceptance in Parts Work

Richard Schwartz's system is so down-to-earth and understandable, it's easy to overlook its depth and meaningfulness. If you get too focused on its steps, you might lose touch with what I think is its greatest lesson: a deep empathy for each part's *unique emotional issues* and how they originated.

If you can't imagine feeling genuine caring and empathy toward a troublesome part of a client's personality, please keep trying. Don't get hung up on whether these inner parts are actually "real." Tolerate your uncertainty and don't feel foolish talking to and about them as if they exist. Whether they're truly real or not, their effects certainly are. As each of these parts appear, your attitude and approach toward them matters a lot; they will experience you as either shaming or welcoming, so strive for the latter. Your client is watching how sincerely you interact with their parts. After all, if you can take an "imaginary" part of themselves so seriously, they will feel safer sharing more of their inner world with you.

Honoring Parts as Real

Most of us recoil from intense or embarrassing parts of ourselves and try our best to keep them hidden. When someone like you—as therapist—comes along and recognizes those parts' dignity and purpose, and wants to hear from them, it releases tension from the entire personality system. With your encouragement, your client can relax and let these parts of themselves speak honestly at long last. It feels so good to finally let them speak their experience, and it can be incredibly healing. But only as long as you the therapist treat this as-if experience with absolute seriousness and respect.

If you can't accept the psychological reality of your client's parts, you won't be as effective with this method. If you're having trouble with the concept, think of how you might do play therapy with a child. You would never quibble with them about whether their stories were "real" or not. You would accept their metaphorical play as the perfect way for them to express what is going on inside them and in their families. Since many personality parts do come into being while we're still children, this analogy is not far-fetched. You are interacting with young, isolated personality systems that may have formed out of emotional neglect, relational trauma, or desperate needs for self-protection. These parts have minds and hearts that may think and feel very differently from the adult consciousness of the person who has come to see you.

But even if you're accepting, your client may have a hard time taking it all seriously. They may worry about looking foolish interacting with parts of themselves. They'd much prefer to keep distance by speaking from the third person, so you may have to repeatedly prompt them to speak directly from the part's perspective, using I-statements (Gordon, 1970). When a person uses "I," speaking as the part, it creates a right-brain existential experience that promotes emotional integration more than talking *about* the part. If you honor the reality of a client's parts at all times, it'll help you resist the temptation to think of them as little more than superficial roles or troublemakers. Try to imagine each part three-dimensionally and relate to them respectfully with real curiosity and empathy. They are your client's innermost aspects and are often linked to traumas, so they are exquisitely sensitive to humiliation or dismissal.

Understanding Child Exile Parts

Think of child *exiles* as the personality parts that carry our earliest and most shamed needs and traumas. These are the feelings and self-states that are too painful or embarrassing to sustain contact with. We cope with them by exiling them into unconsciousness or fencing them off into a dissociated state where we try to keep them entirely separate. Feeling so pushed away and rejected, these parts still carry feelings in their original distressing intensity because they haven't seen the light of day long enough to be explored, processed, or integrated. People—and especially their protector parts—have a strong instinct to keep these emotionally devastated parts hidden and secret even from themselves; they're sure they would feel something terrible or shameful if they were exposed.

Parts work gives you and your client a structured way of talking about these parts and relating to them while not being overwhelmed or scared by them. Although the protector parts of the personality keep the exiled parts hidden and unconscious, our therapeutic hope is that one day the person will get to know all their parts and welcome them as valued members of the overall personality, under the leadership of the adult true self.

Nurturing the Exiled Feeling Parts

To get to know an emotional exile part when it shows up, ask your client to describe this upset part, what they look like, how old they are, etc. You and your client can get to know the part by interviewing the part, either through having the client silently ask the part questions and reporting back to you, or by your interacting directly with the part, whichever feels most comfortable to the client.

This gives the client a safe, structured way of getting to know the feelings and agendas of the upset part, while showing the client that this part can be related to in a compassionate and deliberate way by the adult true self.

After hearing from the part, you could ask your client: *"How would you respond to this upset part if it were a real child? What do you think it needs? Can you go ahead and imagine giving that to them now?"* And afterward: *"How does it feel to show caring to this child?"* and *"What's it like to be showing caring to this child in front of me?"* By modeling this compassionate approach, you are offering the client a therapeutic, nurturing template for how to deal with their upset and vulnerable childlike inner parts, not just in the session but anytime in the future. By asking them how it feels to be doing this in the presence of the therapist, you are building emotional intimacy and strengthening their awareness of themselves as compassionate and caring.

Blending and Merging by Parts

Sometimes unintegrated, unconscious child-parts of ourselves take over in a moment of distress. IFS doesn't see these takeovers by parts as intentional, pathological, selfish, or immoral, but as a natural response to feeling triggered or overwhelmed. Everyone falls back on the automatic maneuvers from childhood that have protected us best. But in therapy we can work with those parts to bring them under the leadership of a wiser adult self that can see the big picture and choose more reasonable and adaptive responses.

Exiled parts cause the most problems when they take over and suddenly merge with the main consciousness of a person's personality. When there's *merging* or *blending* by a part, we are not just *aware* of an inner part, we *become* that inner part (Schwartz, 1995). It might be a traumatized child part; or a defensive protector part; or a relief-seeking firefighter; but whichever it is, it steps in and we see only through its eyes. We entirely lose touch with our true self and adult perspective. We are swept away by extreme feelings, such as getting distraught, overreacting, or helplessly watching ourselves do and say things we know we may regret later. When merged with our most emotionally injured parts, we can instigate some of the most damaging encounters of our lives.

When we blend with a part, we rarely notice it's happening. We think we're still in our main consciousness, but we're not. All of us have the potential to be taken over by a part and start acting out its agenda, even if it could be self-defeating or harmful. This is particularly true with self-criticism and self-attack. We think it's normal to be upset over making mistakes, when really we are in the grip of a protector part that thinks we'll be safer if we beat ourselves up over every misstep.

Emotionally coercive EI parents demand submissiveness from their children—forming parts that live in shame, guilt, self-doubt and even fear. Protector parts approve of such self-negating feelings because they know that these reactions pacify the EI parent. Shame, guilt, and fear can turn into anxiety attacks, depression, or other symptoms later in life, as these parts continue to think self-criticism and inhibition are needed to maintain security and stability—even years after growing up and leaving home.

Clients can regain self-leadership by learning the signs of being merged with a part, such as compulsive self-criticism or overwhelming feelings, such as abandonment, rage, or worthlessness. Mergers with a wounded part are usually accompanied by despair about things ever getting better. In fact, anything that seems terrible or like the end of the world is probably a childhood part speaking.

Alerting clients to these unconscious takeovers gives them the option of unblending from these panicky, regressed parts and moving back into relationship with their more adult, more objective self. A person who understands how and why merged parts take over can attend to the needs of that reactive part, rather than acting out its past traumas in present day encounters.

Lead with empathy before interpretation Focus on feelings before doing parts work. Before addressing the merger with your client, first fully receive their part's feelings, taking them completely seriously and validating their legitimacy with: *"Of course you feel that way."* That instant acknowledgement calms the part immediately. By unequivocally affirming the truth of the child part's emotional experience, you show your client that they're in safe hands. Welcoming and relating directly to this inner child part's feelings creates the deepest levels of rapport, acceptance, and healing.

Pointing out the takeover At some point, *after listening deeply* for a while—and especially if the client stays acutely distressed and is having trouble settling—you might suggest that it seems like a child part may have merged with the client right now, swamping them with its pain. Once your client gets the idea of being taken over by a part, it can help them regain self-connection and self-possession. To that end, you or your client can ask the distressed part to separate and step back to give you a little room to converse with it and find out what's been triggered. You might say something like this to your client:

> *It feels like maybe a child part of you has taken over and merged with you—like when someone drowning latches onto the person trying to save them and tries to crawl on top of them to get their head above water. This panicky part is not helping you right now. See if you can ask this part to move back and give you some room, so we can talk to it and find out what's wrong. Ask it to do that now, and tell me when it has moved back.*

You can use this approach any time you experience a client getting overwhelmed by or stuck in intense emotion, especially if your empathy doesn't seem to be calming them.

Richard Schwartz (1995) discovered that merged parts will respect these requests, stepping back from blending with the client when asked so you can work with the feelings in a less overwhelming way. When you are in communication with the part, it stops trying to take over because it's getting what it needs: serious attention from someone. Sometimes these intense emotions have recent origins, but more often these are traumatized parts whose feelings were split off and banished in childhood and now are grabbing the chance to be heard.

Getting Permission from the Protector to Proceed

Working with protector or manager parts is actually much more common than discovering child exile parts. Protector-work often makes up the bulk of therapy, since they're often behind symptoms, avoidances, and what looks like from the outside like self-defeating behavior and relationship problems. Experiencing the pain and fear of exile parts can be intense and riveting, but understanding and working with protectors is the focus for changing self-defeating life patterns.

The dramatic emergence of strong exiled emotion in a client can make you as therapist feel that you're getting somewhere in therapy. While it's essential to support and attend to the emerging feelings, you don't want to try to elicit or encourage strong emotion until you have created an atmosphere of total safety in the therapy (Fosha, 2000). Keep in mind that if you jump in and start opening up the feelings even more, you are running the risk of alarming a client's protector-part whose sole mission is to keep these raw feelings suppressed. With any abrupt forward movement, watch out for blowback from an alarmed protector part.

This insight from IFS explained something that I had witnessed in therapy. Once, a client had a very emotional, cathartic session with me, making it seem that finally we were making great strides. To my horror, she returned the next week reporting that she'd had an awful week, feeling more depressed and anxious than ever. This made no sense to me since I thought her catharsis would've helped to alleviate these symptoms.

But from the point of view of my client's subconscious protector part, we had let an exiled, out-of-control child part break through, violating the protector's mission of keeping these traumatic emotions under wraps. So the protector fought back against the therapy, shutting down my client with worsened symptoms, as if to say "There'll be no more of *that!*"

There was a simple solution to this, but I didn't know it at the time. When you get to something difficult and deep, leave enough time at session's end to check back in with the protector to see how it's feeling about letting these feelings become conscious. For instance, you could say to the client: *This has been a very important session, you really dealt with some big things. But before we finish for today, can we check in with your protector part to see how it feels about this?*

Then you can either speak directly to the protector, or ask the client to check in with it, asking, *Was this session okay with you? Did anything make you nervous? Are we moving too fast?* Even if the protector seems fine with it, it's still a good idea to reassure the protector that you are aware of its concerns, reaffirming that you want to know if the work ever feels threatening to it. Establishing a deliberate partnership with the protector and seeking its permission to proceed saves time in the long run and avoids iatrogenic regressions from overly ambitious sessions.

Talking directly to protectors like this has an emotional immediacy and integrating effect that doesn't occur with intellectual interpretation. Imagine if, instead of engaging the protector, you interpreted to your client that they were defending against their feelings or afraid to get better. Your client would feel implicitly misunderstood because they know that something other than their conscious mind took over, something with a will of its own—it wasn't *their* defense or fear, it was something *apart* from them. By giving the protector part its due as an autonomous part of the personality, your client doesn't have to take the uneasy (and erroneous) responsibility of accepting the defensive behavior as their own.

Left to themselves, protectors see no need to change anything. They found their solution in childhood, set it up as a repeating pattern, and never went back to check whether it was still a good idea. As such, the protectors in your client's personality will likely rise up against suggestions for change or growth as foolhardy and dangerous.

By listening to the protector's worst fears about what such opening up might mean or lead to, you create an opportunity to reassure the protector about your constructive motives. You explain that you're trying to defuse these pent-up feelings, so they cause fewer problems later on. Your client's protectors will only trust you to do your work if they feel safe in your consideration of them and their protective mission. The protector has zero interest in your client's self-realization or growth; it's still fixated on trying to survive the original childhood emotional environment.

Bringing Protectors Up to Date

Protectors don't learn by themselves that growth and new opportunities are not dangerous or threatening. We have to point it out to them. They couldn't care less about learning or updating their perceptions; they're only worried about the next threat. Frozen in time, they don't even realize that we've grown up and become a capable adult. For them, we're still a helpless child who needs their interventions. So, as Schwartz suggests, it's worth asking a protector how old they think your client is, and then informing them of their real age and adult status. This usually comes as a surprise to the protector and helps unburden them from feeling the sole responsibility for keeping your client safe.

Similarly, after an especially intense or emotionally open session, it's worthwhile to take a moment and point out to the protector that the client opened up, shared their feelings, and *nothing bad happened*. No one was hurt, no parent was shocked, no harm occurred as a result of their openness. Without this explicit reassurance, the protectors would never notice this on their own. After all, they are programmed to protect; not notice when things change. You must draw it to their attention if they are ever to realize it at all.

The protector part needs your reassurance that you aren't potentially exposing your client to attack from authority figures. Those feared authority figures could be actual people in the outside world, but they could also be internalized of EI parents and authorities who live on eternally in your client's inner world.

Protectors see increased autonomy as a very dangerous development that could create an imminent threat to your client's safety. Your job as therapist is to make your client aware of this protector resistance so that your client's reasonable true self can take it into account and have the final word on which way the person's life should go. When you work considerately with the wary protector parts and empathize with their concerns, protectors feel safer to be more collaborative as your client moves forward. If you don't respectfully take the protectors into account, they'll defeat you, because to them you'll seem reckless instead of helpful.

Countertransference and Parts Work

If we as therapists get emotionally reactive to a client, we may have been triggered into countertransference issues from our own childhood. Perhaps the client's behavior triggered us into old vulnerabilities of feeling rejected or shamed. As a result, we might feel a strong urge from our inner protector parts to defend and close ourselves off emotionally.

But we can keep our internal drama safely contained if we stay in touch with our protector parts. With the advantage of parts understanding and our resolve to stay in our true self as much as possible, we can avoid worsening things with our own reactivity. (Our client's defensiveness always holds a hidden gift for us: it sparks our own self-therapy.) Parts work allows you to be a compassionate observer who recognizes yet contains impulses from different aspects of yourself, thereby keeping a rein on countertransference feelings. In this way, you don't identify with these parts or turn them loose on your client.

Parts Work and Nonjudgmental Self-Caring

IFS helps us realize that our exiled and hurting inner child parts can prompt all kinds of desperate and regrettable behavior. A wise therapist knows that in heated moments, reactive parts usually make conflict and suffering worse. The compassionate therapist also knows that once their ACEIP client reconnects with their true self, they'll feel bad about what they've said or done.

When clients feel ashamed of or rejecting toward themselves for some regrettable behavior, it's an ideal time to do parts work. Guilt and self-recrimination only encourage the client's personality to continue splitting into warring parts that unsuccessfully fight to "get rid" of each another. Rather than letting a client reject themselves, as in "I'll never do that again," you can use this opportunity to say: *"Instead of making a resolution, what if we tried to understand why a part of you felt it had to do that in the first place?"* By engaging your client in curiosity about the part's behavior, you may be able to get to the bottom of the impulse and the motive of the part from which it arose.

IFS-informed therapy is one of the best ways I know of understanding and working with problematic behavior without pathologizing it. Your client learns to show a self-caring kindness toward themselves, as they seek to understand a part's motives more deeply. A therapist familiar with these methods understands that each of the parts needs to be understood from the standpoint of how they are trying to *help* the client, with sympathy for how burdened each part is by its compulsive protective reactivity. Working compassionately with the parts as they arise is a true path to healing, though this may be hard for clients to accept at first.

The Wish to Get Rid of Parts

Once an ACEIP client learns about parts, and realizes that it is a part that's been causing them problems, their first question is likely to be: "How do I get rid of it?" As the child of EI parents, the ACEIP client has learned to reject any aspect of themselves that might bring criticism or rejection from others. Having been taught to fear disapproval, they cannot believe that difficult or needy parts hold anything good for them or deserve to be part of their personality.

Thus, one of the hardest things to get across to an ACEIP is that we can't get rid of parts of ourselves. Once parts come into being, it helps to think of them as little entities that have to be accommodated, because they are worthy of our attention and, frankly, because they are not going to go away. They come into being for a purpose and don't change until they find a new mission and meaning.

IFS teaches us that our best option is to *transform* these parts by understanding and accepting their motives while trying to find more constructive ways to meet their needs, with fewer negative consequences. We have new goals to offer our ACEIP clients: integration is the goal; living in peace with our parts is the goal; self-knowledge, self-acceptance, and self-leadership overall are the goals. Here's our mission statement to clients: we don't throw parts of ourselves away; we help them.

Your ACEIP clients can think of their personality as a set of Russian nesting dolls, where inner parts hold ever smaller parts, all the way down to the innermost "baby." The goal is to see one's true self as the all-inclusive big doll, containing and maintaining harmony and respect among all the rest who must live together inside.

Putting IFS into Practice

As an example, let's look at what you might say to an anxious, self-critical ACEIP client to start IFS work with their protector parts.

Imagining the Part

To bring the part into awareness, you could say something like:

I'm wondering if you'd be interested in trying something new. I'm thinking that it might help us if we better got to know the part of you that gets so critical toward yourself. If you stand back and picture the part of your personality that criticizes you, what image do you get? What do they look like? How old are they? Do they remind you of anyone you've known? What would be a good descriptive name for them?

Introducing the Part

Next, have your client invite the part to a conversation. You might say: *"Could you ask this part, silently in your mind, if they'd be willing to answer some questions and talk with us today?"* Give your client a chance to make contact with the part, and then ask: *What did they say?"* If the part is not willing to talk, be accepting of that, but ask if it would mind telling you why. Express your understanding of its position, ask it if it would be okay to try to talk again later, and then drop it. Instead, ask what your client thought of the part, having them speculate on what they think that part might be trying to do for them.

If the part *is* willing to talk, you can suggest questions for the client to silently ask the protector part. If your client is willing to interview the part, you can suggest nonconfrontational questions for them to ask the protector to understand what it's trying to accomplish with all the self-criticism, and why. If it gets too clunky with the client translating everything back and forth, you can ask to speak directly with the part. Sometimes conversing with the part directly is the more emotionally intimate approach, allowing you to forge a direct working relationship with that aspect of your client.

To take this more direct approach, say to your client: *"I wonder if it would be okay to speak directly to the part of you that makes you feel really bad about yourself when you've made a mistake?"* If your client is okay with this, ask your client to step aside psychologically and let the protector part speak through them to talk with you directly. Always remember to tell your client you'll be sure to let them know when the exercise is finished. Don't leave them wondering how long they have to step aside to let the protector speak.

Say, for example: *"Okay, now let's invite this self-critical protector part to come forward in your mind."* Pause for the transition and then introduce yourself.

Establishing an Agreement with the Part

Since protectors often require negotiations before they cooperate, let's look at the first steps of establishing a therapy relationship with them. If your client is willing for you to speak directly with their protector part, here's how your conversation might go with a self-critical protector.

> *Thanks so much for being willing to talk with me today about* [client's name]. *You're the part that makes sure* [client's name] *becomes very self-critical whenever they make a mistake?* (Wait for acknowledgment.) *First of all, I want you to know that I appreciate all you've done for them over the years. I know it can't have been easy to make sure that they always evaluated their behavior and worked to make as few mistakes as possible. You must have had to be very vigilant all the time, right?* (Wait for acknowledgment.) *I know what hard work that must have been, and how much you must care about them to be doing this job. I just want to thank you for all your dedication and caring.*
>
> *I imagine you must get very tired at times. I was wondering if you could tell me why it has been necessary over all these years to point out* [client name]*'s mistakes so quickly and make sure they feel really bad about them?*

From here the discussion is going to take its own turns, but your attitude should remain one of civility, curiosity, and 100 percent respect to the protector's point of view.

When you have listened to the protector's logic and feel like you understand its point of view, you can wrap it up by saying something like:

> *I understand. You have been doing a tremendous job on* [client name]*'s behalf for a long, long time. I know that you only want the best for them and have given up a lot of other activities that you might have enjoyed simply in order to help them improve themselves and stay safe. I want you to know that I see what you've been trying to do, and I for one am deeply grateful for your efforts all these years.*

When this is done sincerely, the protector part often becomes emotional over finally being understood. Then, following Richard Schwartz's protocol, say something like:

And I want to ask you something: If [client's name] and I could find another way to keep them safe and motivated to improve themselves that didn't require you to be so critical of them, would you be willing to step back and let us try that? If I promised that we would never do anything that could get them in trouble or make things worse?

Would you be willing to let us try? I'm not asking you to take my word for it. It's on us to prove to you that the new way will cause no harm. You could step back in and resume any time if you didn't think we were doing a good enough job.

Meanwhile, you could be thinking about what else you might want to be using your energies for. If you didn't have to spend so much energy pointing out their mistakes, what else might you prefer to be doing?

The protector might decide that, for instance, it would like to retire from relentless self-criticism, but might enjoy still using its eagle eye for constructive performance review or quality control tasks. Or perhaps it would like to take up art, music, or a foreign language: something that requires attention to detail but much less anxiety. Or maybe it just wants to get to be a child again and see what each day brings. Each protector has different preferences for retirement.

Unburdening the Parts

IFS sees both protector and exile parts as carrying too much pain and responsibility on their young shoulders. These parts come into being in response to injury and carry burdens of suffering and defensiveness from the past. IFS offers an *unburdening* ritual in imagination that asks a client first to identify the burden carried by the part—for instance, endless negativity and hypervigilance in the case of a self-critical part. You can invite your client to help that part eliminate their outdated, burdensome beliefs and behaviors by imagining annihilating these fear-based burdens, using natural elements, such as wind, water, fire, burial, or any other metaphorical form of clearing that comes to them.

However, don't get this confused with trying to get rid of the part itself, which is not possible. You are only trying to relieve the burdensome childhood *mission* that the part has been carrying. The part and its energies still exist, but hopefully are free to start over with more rewarding goals. (Please see Richard Schwartz's material on IFS if you're interested in finding out more about this particular technique [1995, 2021, and https://ifs-institute .com/].)

While I sometimes use this imaginary ritual of unburdening, I've found that ACEIP clients seem to naturally unburden themselves and their inner protectors once they realize that their original mission no longer fits their adult life. However, shared-imagery exercises like the unburdening ritual are worthwhile because they can strengthen your ACEIP client's use of metaphor and right-brain imagination, not to mention giving you both a shared memory of working together to set them free. The imagery exercise may or may not be the operative event that actually frees them but doing it together in imagination creates a supportive memory that strengthens your therapeutic bond, especially if you make a point to ask them afterwards how it felt to do that with you.

Protectors Censor "Dangerous" Thoughts and Feelings

Protectors are not just guarding against *behaviors* that threaten the status quo; they are on the lookout for "dangerous" *thoughts* or *feelings* too. Remember, protectors come into being when we are still children, often while we're still in the grip of a preschooler's magical thinking. It seems to children that grown-ups can read their minds, and they may even be told that God and Santa Claus know what they're thinking and feeling. If your ACEIP client has been shamed or retaliated against by parents just for their feelings or thoughts, it's no wonder their protectors fear that others will see through them even before they've actually done anything.

Some of the most impactful moments in therapy with ACEIPs are when you encourage clients to pause and tune in to their true thoughts and feelings, even if they are embarrassed or afraid to. As discussed above, when feasible, it's always best to check with the protectors as you do this, so that reflexive guilt and fear don't boomerang and make things worse.

Taking the example of a difficult EI parent, you might ask your client: *"Just pause there for a moment, that minute right after you hung up with your mother—what were you feeling in that split second?"* Or you could say: *"Tell me what you thought right after your father said that thing about your career."* If they share a negative thought or feeling they had, that's a good sign of their willingness to trust you with an uncomfortable emotional truth.

But they may also express self-criticism or shame over telling you what they really felt and thought. If so, it's a golden opportunity to explore why they feel this way even in the privacy of their therapy session, when it's just the two of you. Rather than reassuring them that there are no bad thoughts or feelings, instead explore with them what *their protector* thinks about such thoughts. You may find the protector part believes these thoughts are betraying the EIP, or that others will somehow find out about them.

When a client allows themselves the mental freedom to have the thought—or the emotional autonomy to express their real feelings—it means that they are beginning to feel entitled to have their own private experiences free and independent of their EIP. This is a milestone event in therapy, because their protectors have apparently accepted that it's safe for your client to feel their real feelings and think their true thoughts, because no one can read their mind. They're an adult now, and they can keep their thoughts to themselves if they want to.

Strengthening the Sense of Self

Helping your client to practice being honest with themselves about their true inner experiences is also a powerful exercise to strengthen your client's sense of self. Finally feeling free to have their own private reactions contributes to your client's secure sense of being an individual—and one who may be very different from their family members or loved ones. The self has privacy to grow once your client's protectors realize that admitting their true thoughts and feelings to themselves—or telling their therapist—is not betraying or insulting anyone. It is a totally private experience that every adult is entitled to.

Parts Help Explain the Healing Fantasy

The concept of parts also helps explain the origin of healing fantasies about how their EI parents might one day change and treat them with genuine interest, love, and respect. Think of the healing fantasy as coming from a hopeful child *part* in your client that believes in magic and wants to believe that the parent can change, even if their adult mind knows better. Child parts need to believe parents will change, that they'll find a way to unlock the parent's heart. Seeing the healing fantasy as a child part's dream will increase your client's empathy for their younger self. It can bolster your empathy too. It's easy to get impatient with the lingering hold that EI parents seem to have over their adult children, but it becomes much easier to work with when you realize you are dealing with a child aspect of your client's psyche, not their reasonable adult self.

For instance, consider the difference between these two ways of pointing out that your ACEIP client has unrealistic hopes for changing their parents:

- *"You seem to be holding on to a childlike hope that one day you'll be able to get your parents to change."*

- *"There seems to be a childhood part of you, an inner child, who still has hope that one day their parents will want to change."*

As a client, which statement would make you feel more hopeful about your own capacity to change? Personally, I would prefer to hear that it's a *part* of me that is clinging to the unrealistic hope, because then I can work with it as a separate part of myself, like a disappointed child, that needs my special attention. I wouldn't feel embarrassment over the implication that I was childishly chasing an illogical or impossible goal. The first phrasing has a tone of confrontation—even if it's said kindly. The second phrasing elicits empathy and hope of change, plus compassion for the child part's innocent motive.

By identifying the healing fantasy as a childhood reaction to distress or deprivation, we easily understand why the part clings to it. Children need hope to grow, and they need to have faith in their ability to one day change their parents, or else despair might gain a foothold. Children have too much growing to do to become brutal realists or to give up on their perceived ability to change their world. It's part of the resilience of childhood to always believe that things could get better. Magic and miracles help us to get through hard times over which we have no control.

The EI Parent's Moments of True Self

Finally, we can use IFS parts work to understand that while most EI parents interact defensively from their protector parts, once in a while they—like everyone else on earth—operate out of their true self. During such moments, they might show fleeting empathy, be understanding, or back down from a rigid position. They seem different and more accessible, and they are. They are temporarily present and aware of their child's feelings.

The child part of us sees this as proof that a good parent is "in there" somewhere, behind the fortress walls, if only the child could coax them out. The ACEIP's child part is sure that there must be a way of keeping the parent in that ideal state. All the child knows is that for a moment they caught a glimpse of what it would feel like to have their parent be emotionally available. They believe there must be a way of conjuring that again, if the parent would only try. Your job as therapist is to appreciate the innocent desire to reach that parent, but also to help your client help their child part to accept that they simply can't *make* another person be different.

Nevertheless, more satisfying interactions with their parent might be possible through their own individuation efforts. By keeping a strong, conscious connection with themselves during each contact, and by being authentic instead of feeling they have to become who the parent wants them to be, your client (in all their parts) can feel much less inhibited in the relationship. They can make sure *something* genuine and congruent happens in the relationship, even if it's only one-sided.

Forming Supportive New Parts

While in childhood we naturally formed parts to handle emotional challenges, as adults I think we can also form newly supportive parts of our personalities that foster our growth and health. For instance, we might feel the comforting presence of a supportive loved one during hard times, or perhaps imagine the voice of our therapist when advice is needed. Thanks to our tendency to internalize our relationships, anyone we admire, have depended upon, or learned about can help us. Or we might merge with a source of wisdom and guidance coming from within ourselves. Reparenting our inner child self (Johnson, N., 2025 [in press]; Hadjigeorgalis, 2024), turning to internalized spiritual figures, or even listening to our own intuitive inner guide are all ways that internal parts work could be used to bolster emotional maturation.

Another example of progress fell in the area of her immediate family. Michelle's youngest daughter was having trouble adjusting in daycare, a situation that in the past would've caused Michelle to feel guilty, embarrassed, and anxious. But Michelle knew her child's personality, and suspected from the teacher's manner that the teacher was responding to her daughter in a rigid and detached manner, preventing her daughter from establishing a bond. As Michelle put it, "This time I didn't shut down. I just handled it. Today's my daughter's last day there. Screw what everyone else thinks, this is her. I know her, this is what this is about. I didn't take the bait this time to spiral into 'What's wrong with her?' or 'Am I a bad mother?' I could see what was happening."

Finally, Michelle reported an instance of being unusually effective at work. In her human resources job, she'd had to confront a senior manager about her bullying and intimidating behavior toward junior employees in meetings. Michelle had received several complaints about this woman, and the office morale was being affected. "I was really anxious before I did it, but I didn't avoid it," Michelle reported.

I could tell from her tone of voice that she was pleased with herself about this meeting, so I told Michelle, "I want to hear about what you said that made you feel proud of yourself." I wanted to keep the focus on validating and spelling out her successes so they could be more consciously incorporated in her self-concept. Here is Michelle's analysis of the meeting.

> I was able to objectively observe what she was doing and not let her take over. One way or the other, I was going to tell her what I wanted to say. I saw the bigger perspective, plus I knew I was going to document her response, so I had the attitude, I'm just going to see what she does. The reality was very clear. My biggest shift was that my primary goal wasn't to make sure she stayed calm—like it would've been in the past. My motivation was not to appease her, or make sure she didn't get upset, or help her to regulate herself. I don't think I've ever had such a direct confrontation with an older female like that. I didn't let her out of it. I accepted that she didn't mean to upset anyone, but I stayed connected to myself and presented the reality to her that she still had made the younger staff feel intimidated.

In each of these transformational situations, Michelle was describing her stronger sense of self ("I feel more alive, and more living in line with my true self"). Based on increased confidence in her own experience, she was sure of what she felt, what she had observed, which was the right way to go, and why. She was pleased and proud of herself for acting from the promptings of her own deeper knowing.

These incidents showed Michelle had transformed into a person who was confident in her perceptions and wasn't going to dismiss her own instincts and what she knew was right. Instead of worrying about what others thought of her (a very common symptom of untreated ACEIPs), she was honoring her own experience and acting accordingly. Michelle knew her feelings and needs very well by this point; no one was going to blindside her by shaming her or pulling rank. She was now in touch enough with her true self that she trusted her ability to understand the reality before her.

This kind of transformation is possible when ACEIPs, due to their increased self-awareness and self-trust, can reject psychological pressure from others and stay true to their own needs and feelings. Michelle, like many other successful ACEIP clients, now listened to her own inner guidance and sense of self independent from EIPs. She was no longer willing to unquestioningly accept their authority and distortions of reality. Michelle hadn't just changed her thinking and behavior: her view of herself and her place in the world vis-à-vis other people had undergone a transformation.

Recognizing Self-Change

You'll notice that Michelle was very aware of how her viewpoint had changed since she started therapy. From the very beginning, we always took time to explore and analyze her responses to any situation that caused her stress or anxiety, no matter how small. Whenever I detected self-confident changes in her responses, I would always reflect this to her, and soon she got in the habit of noticing these shifts within herself. Michelle had learned a lot about herself, especially the way that authority figures could at times make her cringe and doubt her own decisions and boundaries. Therefore, she really noticed the difference when she no longer felt paralyzed by others' potential disapproval or disagreement.

Michelle had to develop a sense of her own self and confidence in her judgment before she could interact with authority figures with more equanimity. To do that, she had to know her own emotional truth, moment to moment. The difference for her came when she realized that she had the right to speak up for what she felt was right, and that others did not have the right to overrule her as if they were the most important person in the relationship. Now it no longer seemed outrageous or impertinent for her to have her own goals and point of view.

Noting, Reflecting, and Supporting Growth

Any time you comment on your client's psychological growth, you make it real to them. As you see more evidence of their self-development, you can enjoy pointing out to them these signs of their progress. Often people change before they notice that they've changed. For example, in response to Michelle's descriptions of her transformed experiences, you could say something like:

- I'm just noticing how clear you were with yourself about what you wanted to do.

- You're really not taking on responsibility for your mom's feelings these days.

- Yes, you knew what's right for your daughter and you could tell what she needs.

- That's right! You weren't going to roll over and let her keep bullying people. You had a job to do and you stuck with it.

Any time you witness your ACEIP client doing something brave or self-affirming, give them the words for it. Remember, your job is not just to foster new strengths, but to help your client incorporate these developments into a more complete and updated self-concept. It's the same thing adequately emotionally mature parents do to help their children form a positive sense of self; they help their child recognize and name their attributes and accomplishments.

When a person realizes how they've changed in their self-awareness, self-trust, and self-reliance, they feel joyful, and proud of their growth. For instance, Michelle now felt more sure of her instincts, confident in her individuality, and able to integrate both emotion and intellect.

Let's look at therapy methods that I've found to be especially helpful in connecting clients with their emotional truth and deeper self-knowledge, thereby building their confidence in their own inner guidance.

Emotionally Focused Therapies

Both Accelerated Experiential Dynamic Psychotherapy (AEDP) (Fosha, 2000; Iwakabe et al., 2020) and Emotionally Focused Individual Therapy (EFIT) (Johnson, S. M., 2019; Spengler et al., 2022) are extremely useful therapy systems to help clients experience and understand their emotional experiences. I'm going to share with you the aspects of these therapies that I have found most helpful for ACEIPs, but I encourage you to explore these models directly for additional ideas yourself.

Emotional Self-Awareness

People who are aware of their emotions have a direct pipeline to their sense of self. Emotions are the most elemental signals we have about our needs, true interests, and all-around safety. When emotions are welcomed and understood for their ability to tell us what we need or what's bad for us, they increase our self-awareness and strengthen our individuality.

Opening Up to Emotional Self-Awareness

EI parents often react negatively to children's intense emotions and impulsive way of saying whatever they're thinking. Their children thus learn to worry about being disapproved of just for being themselves. Having felt rejected for showing their true feelings, ACEIPs learn to defend against their emotions. They get good at denying or minimizing their feelings by intellectualizing and rationalizing them away, using psychological defenses that emotionally disconnect them from themselves. Consequently, the ACEIP's access to their emotional truth and deep sense of self is often blocked and needs help reemerging. As therapist, you can sense the first whiffs of emotional truth and slow things down enough that your client can make that connection with their true self.

Spotting Defenses

To identify defenses, notice when a client shies away from straightforward communication with you. When a client clams up or their communication becomes more impersonal and generalized—e.g., by speaking in an intellectual, vague, superficial, second person ("You feel that…"), third person ("Everyone feels that…"), or philosophical tone ("Life is…")—you can redirect with an invitation to head into deeper waters. In my experience, ACEIP clients appreciate it when their therapist doesn't let them off the hook and encourages more personal, forthright communication. It can feel extremely validating when someone cares enough to pin them down about what they really feel.

Neither client nor therapist enjoys avoiding meaningful content for an entire session. You can invite deeper engagement by saying something like:

> I feel like there's something you want to say, but it's covered with [so many words/so much silence] that I can't hear what it is. Could you use plain, fourth-grade language and just tell me what you really felt in that situation? Let's take a moment and see if you can connect more with what that experience was like for you. I'm really curious.

When the client finally gets so basic and clear that it stirs your empathy and gives you a vivid sense of what happened at an emotional level, you have found your connection. The more you gently challenge their defenses against being known, the more you show your interest in them and help them realize that their inner experiences are significant and meaningful.

Don't hold back if you sense there's a part of their story that they're trying not to emotionally connect with. If you think you're picking up on an unspoken feeling that they aren't reporting, express your interest and curiosity, wondering aloud what it was like for them, even if they aren't able to put it all into words the first few times they describe it.

For instance, let's say a client is reporting that their mother becomes volatile when she doesn't get her way, and how upsetting it is to the whole family, children included. However, your client describes this situation in a matter-of-fact way, with little emotion. You might inquire: *"You know, that sounds like it would be tough to go through, yet you're reporting this very calmly. I wonder what it was like inside you as your mother was doing that. I'm thinking it would be quite upsetting."* Now you have two interesting things to explore: their actual feelings when Mom blows up at everybody, and why they try so hard not to show any emotion about it.

Fuzzy Feelings Are the Beginning

Before they can specifically name their feelings, clients may only be vaguely aware of what Eugene Gendlin (1978) has described as their *felt sense*, a generalized, internal bodily sensation that is a somewhat diffuse but honest first "read" on how an experience feels to us. Think of it as a whole body, right-brained, inner-outer "take" on our entire response to what it feels like to be alive in what is happening right this second. It is sometimes experienced as a kind of energy sensation, especially when it comes to being either energized or depleted by a person or situation (Gibson, 2000). Energy sensations in the body are often expressed in the polarities of feeling attracted, uplifted, and hopeful, versus feeling repelled, drained, or depressed.

Learning to tune in to our overall body and energy sense—our gut feeling—is our most important step in self-awareness, since we sense things emotionally and bodily *before* we can put them into words. While our verbal brain likes to discount our wordless felt sense, our embodied feelings actually do a much better—and certainly faster—job of alerting us to essential cues in our environment. Due to its lack of words, emotional and somatic-experiential knowing can seem somewhat vague on first appearance, but that doesn't mean that its message isn't valid. It's the voice of instinct—our body's neuroception (Porges, 2011, 2017)—that's forever paying attention to the things our left brain might talk us out of. The left brain tricks us when it says that the only thing worth knowing is what we can define consciously.

To further narrow down and articulate the elements of your client's felt sense, you can use trauma specialist Peter Levine's (1997) technique of Somatic Experiencing. (I encourage you to check out the exercises in his book on healing trauma [Levine 2005/2008].) Some clients are baffled by body-focusing exercises and find them hard to take seriously, but it's all part of reconnecting them with their inner experiential world to increase emotional self-awareness. Even if you get only a little bit of hesitant cooperation, you are making inroads into helping them value their inner world. Somatic awareness and metaphoric expressions bypass left-brain defenses against instinctual emotion. Don't worry if the answers that you get from body focusing are not earthshaking; it's not necessary to keep drilling for something "significant." What is more important is how you're teaching your client to notice body and energy feedback and be curious about and articulate their feelings.

By focusing your clients on their feelings and state of energy, you are helping them to integrate both their right- and left-brain hemispheres by embodying and expressing their emotional experiences more vividly. As your client becomes more familiar with their felt sense, they will find it easier and easier to reconnect with. People with the best vitality and engagement in life have an excellent connection with their felt sense. By experiencing their emotional reactions more consciously and honoring the meaningfulness of their emotions and level of energy, your client's emerging sense of self and self-trust further unfolds. You're telling them: "*Your reactions do make sense: you're not feeling this for no reason; this is telling you something true about reality.*"

To explore fuzzy feelings and unclear issues more deeply, you might say something like:

Yes, you felt "uncomfortable." So we know your feelings and gut sense were trying to tell you something about the situation. Let's just pause a moment and see if we can put it into words. Would that be okay? Great. Just focus inward on the feeling, that felt sense you had. Say hello to it [Cornell, 1990]; invite it to get clearer. Be open to any memories or thoughts it brings to you, whether they make sense or not. What was the feeling like? What prompted that feeling?

The key in this exercise is for you to encourage any client effort toward emotional, bodily, and energetic self-awareness and treat it as interesting and potentially revealing. When clients get closer to the heart of the matter, they often experience a spacious "aha" sensation and a feeling of release. As you help them translate their vague felt sense into more specific words of conscious knowing, your client's fuzzy feeling can now become more conscious, verbalized, and integrated into their overall self-understanding. Something about the felt sense will always remain ineffable, but we support and relate to it better through scaffolding it with at least a few words.

Searching the Past for a Similar Situation

Usually just tuning in to the true feeling is enough to give your client a piece of themselves back. But sometimes there's more to a feeling's message. You can further process the feeling by searching for its roots in the past. You can ask your client to scan their past for similar feelings and see if they lead to an old storyline.

Kira's Story

Kira was facing a crisis of confidence following her promotion at work. In her new position, she was invited along on after-work get-togethers and team-building exercises, which she had been looking forward to being included in for years. To her consternation, she became almost panicky the first few times she was invited, finding herself barely able to be social even though the people were friendly and inclusive. Rather than getting frustrated with herself, I suggested that she slow down and give herself time to explore her feelings.

The first thing Kira noticed was the mismatch between her feelings and the other people's obvious acceptance and liking of her. Why was she so afraid of being with them? She liked being around them and felt welcomed and respected by them at work. But whenever they went out after work, it was intensely uncomfortable for her. Kira could feel the feeling but had no idea where it was coming from. (If Kira had been by herself, she could've gone deeper into this through spontaneous, free-associational journaling.)

I asked Kira to continue to hold the feeling in mind, but this time I described the situation out loud in an abstract, boiled-down way to see if it reminded her of anything similar from her past. "Okay," I said. "You're invited along with fun people that you really enjoy being around, and yet you feel really scared.

"Now let that remind you of a similar situation in your past," I suggested. (Try to give open-ended prompts or questions rather than yes-or-no queries such as, "Does that remind you of anything from your past?")

Kira paused, and soon became emotional. In a small-sounding voice, like a little girl, she said, "After my parents' divorce, that's how I felt every time my dad asked me to come do something fun with him. My mother was very angry and depressed and I couldn't wait to get away from her, but it felt like looking forward to going with him was a betrayal of her. He wanted to be with *me*, but he had left *her*. I don't think I could ever let myself fully enjoy those times with him. I knew it would kill her if she ever found out how relieved I was to get away from her and how happy I was to be with him."

After making that connection, Kira drew a deep breath and reported feeling much less anxious. Her feelings made sense to her now, and after a bit more processing of how she had not been bad for wanting her father's attention, she no longer dreaded the work outings. If she ever started to get nervous, she compassionately reminded her inner child part that having fun with people who enjoyed her company was not letting her mother down in any way. But most of the time that wasn't necessary, because her childhood fear that enjoying others would hurt her mother was no longer active.

The important thing about this exercise is that we resolved the forgotten trauma of feeling forced to choose between her parents via a *current* vivid emotional experience. This is very different from the classic psychoanalytic approach that might approach the issue more intellectually and verbally through thought associations alone.

To summarize this technique: Kira focused on deeply articulating the feeling itself, which under inquiry reminded her of a tortuous childhood dilemma that was full of conflicting emotions and motives. Instead of seeking an intellectual interpretation of her symptoms, we focused on the experiential quality of her felt sense. The latter allowed her to enter implicit memory through emotional arousal rather than thought associations, and to find the hidden healthy motive in her anxiety symptom: she didn't want to betray, harm, or anger her mother and lose her support.

Why Consciously Processing Emotion Matters

EI parents' overreaction to their children's expressions of individuality often ends up fostering false-self adaptations (Winnicott, 1989/2018) in their children, inhibiting them from feeling, expressing, and receiving validation of their emotions from others.

With the deceptively simple act of being interested in your ACEIP client's feelings, you're starting a whole new upward spiral of transformational affects (Fosha, 2009)—those positive emotional experiences that accompany growth and energize a person to feel healthier and more confident about who they are and what they need. Diana Fosha (2009) describes the motivational force in people which she calls *transformance*—the opposite of resistance—which sparks growth and transformation. Your interest excites your client's motivation toward growth in self-knowledge, instinctual awareness, and the ability to connect with others at a deep level. Your deliberate attention to their emotion reanimates a vital system that had been switched off in them—or nearly so—due to constant exposure to emotionally immature people's dominance and self-absorption.

Developing Authentic Emotional Self-Knowledge

When my clients tell me they have experienced therapy as transformational, it's their renewed emotional and experiential self-awareness and self-trust they're talking about. Finding oneself is too important a need for nature to give us only one chance at it. Healing occurs any time conditions are right. We reinitiate change and growth every time we reconnect with a smidgen of our self-awareness, self-reflection, or emotional receptivity.

Your empathy, interest, and curiosity open a portal to their unique experience, helping their feelings and felt sense become conscious and expressible. Your receptive manner tells your clients: *"This is something we can talk about. Your experience makes sense and we can understand it together."* Emotions are essential self-knowledge; not something to hide from ourselves. When you help your clients find the right words for their feelings, they can become a source of strength, making them feel more whole.

Clients appreciate your gentle help to be honest with themselves; they too want to retrieve these lost parts of themselves. They know you're not just trying to fix their symptoms, adjust their outlook, or lighten their mood. They will want to join with you to find their authenticity, and to interact with integrity instead of burying their true feelings. This is especially true for ACEIPs, who have been taught to equate being a good, nice person with feeling ashamed of their truest instincts and feelings.

Being the "True Other"

Not only does your client experience a deeper, more vital sense of self after processing deep emotion, they also begin to experience you, the therapist, as what Diana Fosha (2000) calls a *true other.* Through their own emotional awakening, they simultaneously view you with empathy as the valued and unique individual you are. This is Fosha's version of Martin Buber's description of the I-Thou experience (1970). They see you now through their own newly emergent and more conscious self, enabling them to appreciate you with feelings of warmth, love, and gratitude for your help.

To experience another person as a true other is not just a nice experience; it creates an amazing feeling of connection for your client, especially if they grew up around EI family members. Your client may be deeply touched by your willingness to go into these emotional places with them with such sensitivity and understanding.

But being seen by your client as a true other might make you a little uncomfortable at first, especially if *you* grew up around EI family members yourself. Their gratitude may be a bit hard to take if you are more accustomed to supporting rather than being supported. But being *happy* about their feelings toward you supports their emerging individuality and improving self-esteem.

Try not to shy away from processing these moments with them. Sometimes direct praise from a client can feel like a spotlight in the eyes, but if ever there was a good reason to get rid of false modesty, this would be the time. When you process their gratitude without minimizing it, they get to experience someone being comfortable with their deep emotion. Successful therapy is a powerful and life-altering experience for anyone; clients often want to make sure you know what you have meant to them.

Their experience of you, the therapist, as a true other is not the same thing as child-like transference, nor is it an idealization of you. They're not being self-effacing in attributing their growth to your help as a therapist. They know they've done their work, but they want to appreciate you too; their gratitude isn't asking to be interpreted or redirected.

It may feel polite or humble to deflect such positive feedback or to minimize your contribution in favor of highlighting the client's prodigious efforts, but don't miss the point: relating to another person as true other is a moment of respect between equals. They know what you've done for them. It's important to hear them out if they say they could not have done this particular piece of work without you. Don't demur; ask them what they mean. (Remember, when faced with a feeling, don't just accept it; do what you can to deepen it.)

Ella's Story

As an example, I was finishing up my work with a client I had seen for a long time. We had worked together successfully and were processing her growth and development over our years together. At one point she stopped and said, "You've been so key, so instrumental in helping me transform my life by getting back to who I actually am. I've learned so many new skills, I'm just feeling so grateful. I feel just really lucky."

At this point, I implicitly accepted what she was saying, but I sensed she had more to say about these feelings. It wasn't time for me to respond to the content yet; it was an opportunity to encourage more expression.

I replied by keeping the focus on her and asking about her coping now and how it's changed. She explained: "If I feel rattled, I find myself pausing and saying, *Okay, what's really going on here? Why am I responding so strongly to this?* I try to settle and reflect on what I'm really feeling right now. I'll wonder: *Why is it hitting me this way?* No knee-jerk response or shoving it out of the way. I just take a pause, like when you catch yourself and realize what's happening. Then maybe I'll journal. It's a slowing down and looking inward and being okay with the yucky feeling, that *sitting in the dirty diaper* you talked about. Now it's just, *Welp, if that's what I need to do, just do it.*

"I just feel a lot more flexible about my responses. Most things don't require that immediate a response. I can respond as a full person and take the time for that. It's like I had a second rearing and I'm equipped to go off on my own now. I had another chance to go through a developmental maturing process. It just feels super transformative. If I were you, I would feel like such a huge accomplishment. You've had such a huge impact and I just want you to know."

Smiling warmly at her openness, I asked her, "How does it feel to be telling me this?" meta-processing the emotional intimacy between us.

"It feels like I really hope that you really know deeply how important your role has been," she said. "I hope there's no ambiguity. I would feel sad if you didn't realize how grateful I am and how much you've helped me. I hope you never doubted for a minute that you did. I want to make sure that's not lost in any way because to me it's a huge transformation. I can just be a better person for other people too. I'm *way* more open to talking to people about feelings and inner experiences. I'm more willing to talk about stuff now and not let it swirl in my head and get all tangled. I feel a little more confident that I can come to the right answer. And if it's not the right response, I can probably fix it. Things aren't usually irreversible. My parents acted like it was a catastrophe if I made the wrong move, but that's not usually the way it is."

"Can you tell me why it's so important to you that I know this?" I said, again returning the focus to her process. (Here, I'm not diverting her praise, I'm going into her experience more deeply—as usual.)

"It's so real and it's so internal. I always knew you were there for me; you had my back. I can feel it and experience it first-person. I want to be sure that when someone does something really good in the world, it should just pay dividends."

At this point I recognized her regard for me as a *true other*, and that her desire was for me to fully receive her experience with me. She was experiencing my meaningfulness to her, and she wanted to make sure I knew what I had been to her. Not my training, but my empathy guided me toward the genuine response she needed from me.

I responded: "I *do* know what I've done for you—probably with plenty of mistakes and omissions—but I sense what it's meant to you because I've been able to feel your transformation. I remember your suffering when you first came in and I remember feeling like 'This shall not pass.' It was like a mandate, like pulling someone from a river and resuscitating them, and that was just the beginning."

That's the beauty of meta-therapeutic processing: the truth was told, the connection was real, and we confirmed our experience of each other. I left the session satisfied that I had let her know I had realized how urgent her need for help was. My genuine sharing was in the service of validating our real connection. She was able to leave the session feeling satisfied that she had succeeded in letting me how I had helped her. That was her urgent gift to me, a true other, from her true self, on this, our last session. I accepted her gift, exploring it with her and incorporating it into the narrative of our relationship. Deflecting her gratitude with modesty or deflection would not have been a true-other thing to do. If she could be so genuine and forthright with me, I could certainly do the same with her. Like all other feelings, your clients' positive feedback must be both explored and accepted for their benefit.

The Importance of Processing Positive Affects

In the example above, my client and I processed very positive feelings about each other. AEDP therapy would say that processing positive affects is just as important as uncovering unhappy and painful feelings (Fosha, 2000, 2009). Some therapies have a kind of brush-clearing philosophy to growth—that if you pull enough debris out of the way, new growth will occur on its own. But in order to become emotionally literate and self-aware, clients need feedback and honest emotional responses to their positive feelings too. It's crucial in therapy to note and accentuate the good feelings that arise when a client is showing signs of growth.

When you explore positive feelings in a deepening way, you're contributing to their strong sense of self, self-esteem, and a well-articulated self-concept. You're seeing them as a true other whose blooming growth, maturation, and abilities you are tracking and recognizing with appreciation. By doing so, you show them how to notice and own their progress, within a context of emotional intimacy that can be expressed and received as the most natural thing in the world.

Here's another example of how mutual processing of successes and positive affects supports an upward spiral of growth and intensified self-trust and self-esteem in your client.

Maya's Story

Maya was a senior architect. She couldn't wait to tell me about her masterful handling of a difficult situation with a junior colleague who had made a significant error and then reacted defensively to her questions about it. Even though her young colleague's irritation and excuses had made things worse with their customer, Maya was aglow with satisfaction over how she handled it with the colleague. Maya's first urge was to criticize and punish the young man for the problems he had caused, but then she realized, *No, he's suffering. I remember this from when I was younger.*

Maya suddenly saw the situation as a teaching moment, not as an excuse to lose her own temper. If Maya had become reactive, the situation could've deteriorated into mutual blame-casting. She sidestepped her colleague's defensiveness and instead offered practical suggestions for how to avoid this mistake in the future.

Maya was proud of how her increased emotional maturity—based on years of learning how to handle volatile family members from a place of objectivity—had paid off in her conscious decision to remain neutral so she could problem-solve. This was especially significant growth because earlier in her life Maya could've competed with the best of them in her emotional dysregulation.

Noting Maya's profound sense of psychological accomplishment, I further explored her positive affect. Her marvelous emotional achievement demanded thorough processing—we needed to give it the same careful attention we would show toward painful or embarrassed feelings.

"How do you feel about how you handled this?" I asked.

"It felt like I was the most mature person in the universe. Like, who *does* this? *Nobody* does this! Hell, yeah!!" We were both laughing.

"I felt so accomplished," Maya said. "I felt like a leader, like *Order is restored in the universe; order will flow forward!* It was a real milestone in my life, I'm not kidding. I know it's because I've been in psychotherapy for 40,000 years, because I can remember what it was like before. I learned from therapy, way back, that you can make a mistake and not be a terrible person."

"How did it feel as you moved past those urges to get angry or confront him for not accepting responsibility?" I said.

Maya reflected: "Now it's like I'm constantly moving forward instead of getting sucked into a pit of lava that—for some reason—everyone else seems to want to get sucked into. I picture myself in a helium balloon: *You're sending me heat? Let me use it to go higher.* Really, I should send my family a thank-you note for getting to watch them go into all these anger-vortices over the years. But I may have graduated from that."

"You know, as I listen to you," I mused, "it comes to me that your response was like a work of art."

"*Yessss!!!*" she said. "It was designed. It was implemented. I played it like a fiddle! I was the Yo-Yo Ma of this moment, and I achieved the best possible result."

"It feels like a miracle," I said, and Maya chuckled in pleasurable agreement. That's how she experienced it, too.

"Why do you think you didn't get angry with the guy?" I asked, further exploring her positive feeling.

"I didn't want him to feel bad. I knew he felt bad for making a mistake, like I used to. I recognized my behavior from younger days. You know, *you* make a mistake and then you get mad at someone *else*. He's young. None of this stuff is the end of the world, and I don't want him to have bad feelings about it. If he doesn't act on my suggestions, that will be another story, but for now it's liberating to handle this differently."

"So how would you describe your approach with him?" I asked, moving her emotional experience into more left-brain analysis for further integration.

"If you make a mistake, you take a breath, and we find a way to fix it. In this office, this is going to be our new policy about mistakes. We admit it, own it, fix it—and deal with the consequences."

"I'm just noticing how directly you're dealing with reality now," I reflected.

"Yes, I was playing it like an orchestra, pulling everything together for a more beautiful result."

"Dealing with a problem like this could bring out defensiveness and power moves, but you saw a complex reality and did what was good for everybody. You made it *transformative* for both you and him."

An even deeper transformation was of Maya's old self-story of herself as a reactive, easily emotionally threatened person. She was remembering her earlier days of reactivity with compassion, honoring the growth and complexity she had now attained as a wiser adult. With such compassion for her previous self, she was also able to see herself in her young colleague. She realized he was a real and imperfect person too, a "true other" flailing about, trying inelegantly to escape guilt and shame at all costs. Maya's well-developed self-awareness allowed her to avoid conflict and to offer him helpful suggestions that I'm sure facilitated his maturation as a person too.

Share Your Genuine Reaction

You can probably sense the joy on Maya's part in this conversation, and our shared enjoyment of how far she'd come. But it's important to note here that my authentic reactions (e.g., "it feels like a work of art," "a miracle," "transformative") truly reflected how I felt.

I had witnessed something beautiful and awe-inspiring in Maya's mature and emotionally skillful response, and I let her know it. There was no therapeutic advantage for me in maintaining neutrality at that moment; this was something for me to feel along with her while keeping the foremost focus on processing her feelings. She got to share and receive validation for some of the most emotionally mature functioning she had ever risen to. It needed to be recognized and celebrated by the person in a special position to know what it meant for her.

Make Their Experience Even More Conscious

Imagine how the session might've gone if I had received Maya's joy as something nice, but not as the masterpiece of emotional maturation it was. What if I had said, "Good for you, that's great!" and stopped there? Such feedback would've been too vague and pat to lay down an anchor on the experience. Her extraordinarily intentional interaction with her young colleague might've registered as a good day, but it would not necessarily have been appreciated as a demonstration of all her years of work in therapy and personal development. It was important for me to bookmark this by finding the exact words for the *significance* of what she was telling me, and to share that with her, along with my own happiness for her achievement.

thought are mainstays of cognitive behavioral therapy (Beck, A. T., 1976; Burns, 1980; Beck, J. S., 2021), but here we are looking for the broader, earlier unconscious structuring of how clients view themselves in life. They have learned a certain reality, but it can turn out to be an erroneous pattern.

For instance, a client describes feelings of frustration that loved ones aren't more considerate or empathic. This is their reality. But is it that? Or is it that they don't step up for what they want, and rarely say no to others? Perhaps based on the client's experience that speaking up only makes things worse, listening may seem like a safer adaptation than self-expression. Or a client might fear setting a boundary with a pushy EIP, convinced that they would be unable to handle the blowback from that person's displeasure. They "know"—based on their past unconscious emotional learnings about interactions—that claiming rights or boundaries won't go well.

In childhood, this client might have learned, "Ah, I get it. I have no rights to my own opinions or boundaries, and everyone else is more important than me." This emotional learning would guide their actions, but probably never be consciously thought or verbalized by your client.

When you as therapist begin to identify these schemas and put them into words, you loosen the unthinking, emotional grip of the belief. Your client then has a chance to step back and be objective, often for the first time, about how they have made sense of reality. Sometimes the old mental models will fade away as soon as they are articulated in the light of day, while others will require dedicated attention. In this chapter, we'll look at how to help dislodge deeper, reality-distorting beliefs.

I'll be sharing with you some Coherence Therapy–informed interventions based on Brian Ecker's and Laurel Hulley's approach to therapy (1996; 2005–2019), as well as Coherence Therapy's *memory reconsolidation* techniques for lasting change (Ecker et al., 2012; Ecker, 2015, 2024). What follows are adaptations of their methods that seem most suited to the needs of ACEIPs. Since this is but a brief overview, you might be interested in further study of these methods, especially if you'd like to understand how predictable brain-change mechanisms operate across different but similarly successful therapies (Ecker, 2024). This approach has the potential to integrate diverse therapeutic approaches under their shared change-mechanism of updating self-defeating mental models through memory reconsolidation.

Symptoms, Schemas, and Emotional Learning

Many well-known psychological symptoms—such as anxiety, depression, panic, emotional reactivity, and others—originated in patterns of perceiving reality that were formed during a stressful childhood. Over time (or instantly, in the case of trauma), we learn what we can expect from other people, and that, in turn, gets translated into what we "know" we can expect from life. When we are learning from emotionally immature adults in childhood, they can teach us errors about reality that negatively affect us and can take years to repair.

Coherence Therapy (Ecker & Hulley, 1996, 2005–2019) sees symptoms as arising from these unconscious *emotional learnings* that helped us adapt to past specific circumstances, especially those that felt stressful or threatening. This experience-based "knowledge" of how life supposedly works is then applied to any current situation that unconsciously resonates with past conditions. A symptomatic episode suggests that an old schema has risen up and taken over—in IFS terms, you might think of it as a protector or child part (Schwartz, 1995)—and your client now interprets circumstances through the lens of a past *emotional truth* that justifies the need for the symptom.

As children, when distressing episodes happen repeatedly, we may mistakenly conclude this is our lot in life. Memories are all we've got to orient ourselves, so your clients might be stuck in emotional templates of reality (schemas) from their childhood, even if these mental models are now self-defeating and symptom-inducing. Such learnings are difficult to change through conscious willpower because many are coded in implicit, unconscious memory. Without exploring how your clients made sense of the world as children, we omit this essential ingredient of memory, which has to be addressed for real transformational change. Our job is to reveal these assumptions, making them more conscious and explicit, while working with the client to understand how they might have come to those conclusions. Old emotional learnings must become explicit before we can evaluate whether they fit our adult life now.

Coherence Therapy prioritizes schemas because they help us decode the underlying *purposes* of symptoms. To the client, symptoms feel alien and unwanted—they're coming to therapy to get rid of them. Symptoms such as depression, anxiety, panic, or phobias often make no sense and interfere with your client's ability to live the kind of life they consciously want. Because symptoms are so much more powerful than reason or willpower, they can make a client feel helpless, undermining their self-confidence and sense of autonomy. Therefore, it helps the client tremendously to find that they do make sense at an unconscious level.

Cognitive psychotherapies teach clients ways of challenging or "counteracting" (Ecker, 2024) their symptoms with top-down, competing thoughts—activating frontal-lobe reasoning to offset emotional reactions—so as to live as good a life as possible. In these therapies, symptoms are seen as misguided and unnecessary behaviors to be modified or controlled. The medical model, in a different language, also pathologizes symptoms as signs of sickness that need external, countervailing cures, like bacterial infections need antibiotics. Removing symptoms is the target of medication therapy as well.

However, the explosion of interest in trauma-informed psychotherapies (Terr, 1990; Herman, 1992/2022; Levine, 1997; van der Kolk, 2014, among many, many others) over the past several decades has spurred a new attitude toward symptoms. Symptoms of trauma, such as dissociation and post-traumatic stress disorder, are now understood as expectable responses to extraordinarily threatening circumstances. Trauma symptoms no longer seem meaningless, like aberrant overreactions, but have been studied down to their physiological roots. A deeper understanding of trauma symptoms and treatment (Levine, 1997; Ecker et al., 2012; van der Kolk, 2014; Maté, 2003) has begun a popular shift away from trying to eradicate the symptom at the surface level toward transforming the underlying "stuck" schema so the symptom can be released as no longer needed for its original protective purpose.

Let me be clear before we go any further that I fully support using cognitive, behavioral, exposure, and medication treatments when they help a person function better and feel more human, especially when the person doesn't have enough resources, insight capacity, or inner strength for more emotionally focused therapies. I see no reason for someone to suffer needlessly when we have rapid treatments that offer some relief. We have all kinds of remedies in our medicine chests that we don't think twice about using to make ourselves feel better. Many times, antianxiety, antidepressant, antipsychotic, and mood disorder medications can give the person back their ability to function, or even be lifesaving. To me, these medications and behavioral treatments can make the difference between being able to enjoy your life and living your life constrained by symptoms. But with clients who can develop insight, I hope to help them transform their underlying schemas to the point where they can automatically live life differently without having to work so hard or rely solely on outside measures.

To sum up: What if the roots of symptoms aren't pathological, but were originally adaptive? What if we understood symptoms as communications from unresolved and frightened parts of ourselves that are doing the best they can? What if symptoms become meaningful once we realize what has happened to a person and how they made sense of it?

Melinda's story

Consider Melinda, an ACEIP who came to therapy for exhaustion and stress over her excessive workload and her inability to relax even when she had the time. She seemed endlessly pushed forward in life as if at the tip of a spear. Using the techniques in this book, we identified her old mental models of reality, originating in emotional learnings, that drove her to work constantly. For instance, I asked Melinda to summarize what she had learned from childhood about being an adult. She said she learned to live "as if people were keeping a clipboard and checking off what I'm doing and not doing." When asked about specifics, Melinda was able to narrow down these "people" to her busy mother, from whom she had a strong desire for approval.

Melinda's mother's history was significant: her mother's mother was an angry, abusive, and depression-prone woman who could become emotionally paralyzed by her dark moods. Melinda's maternal uncle also suffered from depression and had to be hospitalized repeatedly. Melinda's mother solved this dire family pattern with a life philosophy that could be summed up as: "Being in motion is inconsistent with being depressed." Her mother worked all the time, making comments like "If you keep moving, you'll be fine," or "No point in dwelling on the past; move on!" or "If you don't want to end up in a mental hospital, keep busy."

Melinda's mother couldn't allow for reflection or taking care of oneself; in fact, stopping to think or rest was tantamount to inviting mental illness. Now Melinda herself was subconsciously living by her mother's antiquated "technology" for mental health, based on schemas derived from her mother's trauma history. But by bringing her mother's teachings into full consciousness, Melinda could confront her conscious, adult mind with whether this old learning still made sense. For the first time, Melinda made the connection between her driven behavior and her mother's schema for staying mentally healthy—once she did, she could compare realities and make a real choice. Melinda's inherited schema of *work-prevents-mental-illness* could then transform into a conscious embrace of her own need for balance, rest, and recreation.

Our Two Minds See Symptoms Differently

We all live in two realities simultaneously, one constructed by our conscious, reasoning mind and one based on our unconscious mind and implicit emotional learnings. Each mind values different things, and they often disagree about what's important. The conscious mind, centered more in the goal-directed left hemisphere, wants things to be as obvious, certain, and rational as possible. The unconscious mind, centered more in the emotionally attuned, meaning-based right hemisphere, only cares about emotional truth and its needs. As Ecker and Hulley (2005–2019) note, we therapists are always listening to hear from both our client's conscious and unconscious mind. It's like working with two different people at the same time.

When a client is in their *conscious* left-brained mind state, they see absolutely no reason for the symptom they're suffering: it seems pointless, misguided, problematic, and makes them feel powerless. Symptoms are seen as meaningless misfirings, evidence of disorders, pointless products of old conditioning, or errant brain chemistry. From this viewpoint, naturally the client wants to fight against their symptoms, as if they were the enemy.

This mentality of suppressing and eradicating symptoms has governed our psychotherapeutic approaches for a long time.

But as Ecker and Hulley point out, often a client's unconscious mind holds a "prosymptom" stance that secretly views symptoms as *emotionally necessary*, regardless of the client's conscious opinions. Ecker and Hulley articulate the following unconscious prosymptom beliefs of a client in the following quote from their enormously helpful manual, *Coherence Therapy: Practice Manual and Training Guide:*

- "The symptom's existence has deep emotional sense and personal meaning.

- The symptom is at times compellingly necessary for me to *have*, because it is part of *how I avoid an even worse suffering* (italics mine), and so it must *not* simply be stopped or disallowed.

- I myself produce the symptom as part of how I carry out my own urgent purposes (Ecker & Hulley, 2005–2019, p. 4).

From this list, we can see how Melinda unquestioningly accepted her mother's guiding belief for how to avoid familial mental illness. At the time, it did make sense, and it did have deep personal meaning.

Using the Sentence Completion Exercise

Fortunately for psychotherapy, the unconscious mind is like a chatterbox always trying to slip a word in edgewise. If we set up the right conditions, we can arrange for a kind of Freudian slip to slide through a chink in the left-hemisphere wall of words. Coherence Therapy uses an exercise of finishing incomplete sentences to accomplish this. There have been many forms of sentence completion *tests* over the years (Holaday et al., 2000; Rotter et al., 1992; Rotter & Willerman, 1947), but Coherence Therapy makes a *therapy* method out of it with a more informal, interactional approach. This technique is based on the observation that the holistic right brain can't resist jumping in with something true to complete a hanging sentence. Given half a chance, our unconscious mind will smuggle in some truth-telling.

Here's how I have adapted Ecker and Hulley's sentence completion exercise (Ecker & Hulley, 2005–2019, p. 15) in my own words to use with my clients. Tell your clients: *I'm going to say the beginning of a sentence, and then you repeat it after me and finish the sentence with the first thing that pops in your mind. Try not to censor or evaluate it. Just let it come to you. Ready?*

If your client does what most people do and just finishes the sentence without repeating the prompt, praise them and try it again: *Great! Let's try another one; this time repeat the whole prompt and then see what pops in your mind.* Then say the prompt again. (You want a light, neutral tone, to convey that there's no way to fail this.) I've noticed that there's something about repeating the beginning of the prompt each time that seems to pull for more emotional or meaningful content, rather than just letting them free-associate the missing words.

Try each prompt several times. Each time they deliver, appreciate their efforts, and then say, *Let's do it again.* It helps to present the same prompt several times, since with each successive association, the unconscious mind often sneaks through and goes a little deeper. Ask as many or as few different prompts as you like, but when you are done, I recommend picking out one feeling-infused answer that stands out to you, and ask your client to go more deeply into that feeling, telling you what that feeling is like, just as we have done earlier in the feelings work in chapter 7.

Ecker and Hulley (2005–2019) also suggest that you can use sentence completions to get at unconscious interpersonal dynamics by having your client imagine they are talking to a significant other person about the need for keeping a symptom. For ACEIPs, this especially would be someone from their formative years. Now you can use creative sentence completions to get at how certain relationships create a *need* for the symptom (e.g., "*It's important for me to be afraid* [depressed, lose my temper, etc.] *so that I don't/you don't...*") or why *not* having the symptom could be a bad thing (e.g., "*If I wasn't so nervous and afraid, then I/you...*") You can find much more detail in Ecker and Hulley's enormously helpful manual (2005–2019) if this approach appeals to you.

Robert's Story

To illustrate the sentence completion method, let's look at the case of Robert, who was tied up in knots over asking his supervisor for time off from work to take advantage of a trip offer. Robert was in therapy largely due to depression and difficulty in asking for what he needed, so this was an important incident to spend time on. When I questioned Robert about why it was so hard to ask for time off, he replied, "I hate to bother him with what's going on with me"—a classic ACEIP response if ever there was one. At this point I could ask him to explain using his logical left brain, or I could open the portal to the unconscious, emotional dynamics of his right brain with some sentence completions.

After asking Robert what his *feelings in this situation* reminded him of, he explained that while growing up he virtually never talked to his parents about anything personal or emotional, because they so easily turned critical or got upset. I decided to use sentence completion prompts to go into this in more depth so we could access the underlying schemas (emotional learnings) that now dictated his relationships with authority figures. I gave Robert the instructions and here's what emerged.

Therapist:	I agree that when their feelings show up…
Robert:	I agree that when their feelings show up, I will disappear.
Therapist:	(building on last completion) And that way…
Robert:	And that way, their feelings won't get hurt.
Therapist:	When I say my feelings…
Robert:	When I say my feelings, people get hurt and don't like me.

The most remarkable thing about sentence completions is that they usually take you in directions you don't expect. While I was focusing on his overall relationship with his parents, Robert's subconscious mind delivered highly specific truths I hadn't thought to ask about. Robert was afraid of hurting a more powerful person's feelings and of how that might lead to their not liking him anymore. If you are a child, and the more powerful person is your parent, such a risk attains survival stakes at a very primal level in the brain. Asking his supervisor for time off sure didn't seem like it should put his entire source of security on the line, but that was the emotional truth of how Robert felt when dealing with authority figures. We talked about what it had been like for him to keep everything inside so he wouldn't hurt his parents or make them go away.

But what if I had missed this opportunity and instead made suggestions about how he needn't feel like meeting his needs is a bother to people? If I had done that, Robert doubtless would've agreed with me, but he would've felt oddly deflated since I hadn't taken the time to get to *his* truth—his compelling and necessary reasons (Ecker & Hulley, 2005–2019) for not "bothering" people.

After the sentence prompts, Robert's internal schemas and fear of authority figures became even clearer when I asked Robert more about his feeling of something bad happening if he asked for time off.

Robert:	I'm afraid they'll think I'm lazy.
Therapist:	What do you feel when you fear that? (*Note that I didn't ask, "Why do you fear that?" One calls for emotional exploration, the other promotes intellectualization.*)
Robert:	Sad, like I'm a failure. It's a dreadful feeling, like the world is ending in a way. It's a feeling of not being important, being left behind, being alone. Being lost and not knowing how to come out of that.

Therapist: Can you give me a metaphor for this feeling? (*His right brain is activated; he's speaking in metaphors. I want to stay there now.*)

Robert: Like a ship docked at an island. Everyone is getting on, and it leaves, and I see it leaving. People on the ship are looking at me and I'm on the island alone. No one cares and I'm alone. Sitting down in the sand and giving up. They're having fun. Some look back and see me there, but they go on.

Even more poignantly, Robert remembered how he used to channel his feelings of sadness into his teddy bear.

Robert: He had brown plastic eyes. I play with them and hug the bear. It made me want to cry.

Therapist: Tell me about hugging the bear. (*I'm going for the detail that moved me the most.*)

Robert: I made it feel…I was able to turn around and be supportive of the bear…and me. I was taking care of me.

Therapist: And you were crying?

Robert: I was rubbing my finger on his eyes, wanting to cry.

Therapist: You were wanting help and feeling alone. But you were accepting the situation, like "This is what life is like."

Robert: I wanted to take care of someone the way I'd want to be taken care of.

Notice that when I make an empathic guess that's a little off the mark, Robert redirects me to the much more personal and poignant truth. My guess was too intellectual; but no harm done because we're working well together to get the specifics of his feelings correct.

In this dialogue, my attention stays on the feeling and somatic elements of his memory. Whatever touched me most deeply was the next thing I asked about. If I had aligned myself only with Robert's conscious mind, I would have missed the rich material that came out of the sentence completion. By recognizing that all behavior is coherent in some way with a person's underlying mental models from the past, I declined the temptation of trying to urge him out of passivity and instead showed curiosity about his deeper feelings and motives.

Articulating Subconscious Motives

If we were going to help Robert from a cognitive behavioral therapy (CBT) approach, we would expose the fear-based illogic or distorted belief that needed to be challenged. For instance, we might help Robert get to his underlying distorted convictions, such as "opening up leads to rejection" or "bad things happen if I feel too sure of myself." In effect, we could help him re-evaluate and reject his illogical assumptions by exposing these underlying cognitions to the light of reason.

This approach would've offered what Ecker (2024) calls a *counteractive* or *competitive* solution, teaching him how to use his reasoning mind to challenge the illogical or erroneous thought. This top-down approach, using the thinking parts of the brain to challenge the faulty beliefs, is like giving someone a fire extinguisher for a kitchen where little fires break out all the time. Why not try to figure out what is causing the combustions in the first place? (At the same time, good to know where the fire extinguisher is and how to use it.)

Working through Robert's underlying schemas and their associated feelings gave us the emotional reasons sustaining the symptom. Both cognitive and experiential approaches could help him, but one requires vigilance and counteracting while the other creates a transformational shift in the original need for the symptom.

By using the Coherence Therapy approach and other emotionally focused, experiential therapies, we understand our client's symptoms and self-defeating behaviors as long-ago solutions toward safety. Our therapy work becomes more emotional and personal—enabling outdated assumptions to shift automatically. We found the positive, constructive *motive* behind Robert's fear of speaking up, such as, "If I hide my feelings, I can still belong" or "If I stay scared and passive, then worse things [like rejection] won't happen to me."

Approaching his symptoms in this way, Robert didn't have to concede that his expectations were little more than mistaken cognitions. Instead, his anxiety was validated as absolutely justified, given the emotional truth of his childhood situation when he was piecing together his first lessons in life. He wasn't misguided; he was self-protective. On his own, his little-boy part came up with the answer to the problem of EI parents who shied away from any emotional intimacy with him, especially when he was upset. He learned to turn to himself instead and not ask anybody for anything. He even gave himself the comforting he needed, via his faithful proxy, the stuffed teddy bear. Robert was an adaptive genius at an early age.

How to Use Symptom Deprivation

Another way Coherence Therapy tries to uncover the motives behind symptoms is to ask the client to imagine what life would be like if they *didn't* have the symptom. What might happen then? How would their relationships be affected if the symptom went away? Questions like these are designed to project your client into the *lived experience* of a symptom-free future. It works only if you guide the client toward a full affective embodiment of this alternate reality, not just creating a fantasy story in their head.

Anna's Story

For example, Anna was an archeologist who suffered from anxious procrastination and mental blocks every time she had to write up her research findings for a professional journal. Although she had published several well-received articles, she sweated blood every time she reached the downhill part of writing up her research. Now that she was submitting her work to more well-known journals with the potential for wider success, the process had become even more painful. I wondered aloud with her what might happen if she lost the symptom of writer's block and the agonizing struggle that went with it. I asked her to emotionally imagine what it would *feel* like if she just wrote freely and turned out a great article that was accepted by top-tier journals? I was asking her to take away the symptom and see what would happen without it.

Clients always assume that their life would improve immensely without their symptoms, but the beauty of the Coherence Therapy approach of imagining symptom deprivation is that we get specific about what the client *really* believes life would be like if they were free of the symptom. Anna found that when she projected herself into a symptom-free future full of success, she immediately thought of her narcissistic, highly accomplished father and felt a stab of anxiety, thinking about how he would respond.

She responded: "It's like he's the only person who deserves to exist. He's always righteous, and you're supposed to recognize *his* success in life." Anna realized that her father needed to be the star of the family, and that there was a part of her trying to protect his ego by not completing her own work. When I asked how she felt about this realization, Anna said, "Just sad. Very sad. My response is to want to protect him. I even risk hurting myself to do that."

I felt this was no time to soft-pedal things. "No," I said. "You *have* hurt yourself for him, and you're poised to hurt yourself more."

Anna realized that she feared envy and emotional abandonment by her father, not just a refusal to acknowledge her success. "Maybe he wouldn't come unglued, but he would act as if I don't exist. That would be the atom bomb, worse even than him getting angry."

As Anna silently processed this thought, she seemed to become more serious but more peaceful. I asked her what she was feeling.

"I want my work to succeed," she said. "I can't fix my dad. I have to create some joy for myself, and he can share in it or not."

Using Juxtaposition of Emotional Learnings to Change Schemas

Have you ever wondered how your mind selects what to believe out of the tsunami of information that sweeps over it daily? Or how a child gives up magical schemas about the world in order to form an adult perspective? Or how brainwashing (Taylor, K., 2004) can induce a new mental reality that radically alters how a person looks at the world?

The thing that makes humans so uniquely adaptable and endlessly creative is our brain's penchant for dropping outdated information in favor of new ideas that seem to explain reality more accurately. We don't still believe everything we've ever been taught. Much of our old learning is replaced as we come to see things differently. This is what neuroplasticity is all about: the brain changes as we change.

A fascinating technique for change based on this phenomenon is described by Ecker and Hulley (1996; 2005–2019) as *juxtaposition experiences,* a treatment method that has its roots in neurological research into *memory reconsolidation* (Ecker et al., 2012; Ecker, 2015, 2018). This occurs when an old learning (memory) is activated in the face of a new bit of learning that explains reality more accurately. To quote Ecker and Hulley (2005–2019): "In a juxtaposition experience, you are cueing the client to subjectively feel two different knowings concurrently, and both feel real, yet both cannot possibly be true" (p. 47).

When the two learnings, old and new, are juxtaposed in consciousness, the emotionally invested, old learning tends to be overwritten by the new awareness. To accomplish this, Ecker (2015, 2018, 2024) suggests having the client imagine a "split-screen" experience, as if the old learning and the new knowledge are being experienced simultaneously, side by side. With this method, when the old memory is activated and its file is "open," you expose it to new information whose self-evident truth reconfigures its emotional formatting. Even an iron-clad belief or traumatic lesson can become just another thing we used to believe. The old memory is still remembered, like a fact once learned, but its original affective charge vanishes thanks to the new perspective. The person can recall what they used to believe, but now it just seems unreasonable or silly. This unique memory transformation is also showing great promise in new approaches to treating trauma (Trudeau, 2023).

Here's a simple example of how juxtaposition and memory (learning) reconsolidation might work. If you believe that the world is flat, because that's how it looks, and then someone shows you a picture of a spherical Earth from space, while explaining the deceptive straightness of a tiny piece of a curved horizon, you would likely shift your mental model because now the new information makes more sense, explains more data, and is embedded in a whole cosmology of space. Holding the two mental models in mind simultaneously makes it clear which is more likely to be true. This is how we change and grow psychologically. Our brains are designed to divest from old learning as soon as reality convinces us to do so—as long as we don't have psychological defenses that rigidly dismiss or distort reality.

However, a person can eternally defend their status quo by reflexively keeping old beliefs and new evidence separate, just as many EIPs do. For them, their need to be "right" matters more than the evidence. But barring such bullish defensiveness, a person with an adequately mature and integrated mind will subconsciously weigh which interpretation of reality best explains what they're experiencing. You can imagine what an enormous survival advantage that must have given early humans.

As ACEIP therapists, we keep an eye out for these outdated, harmful emotional learnings that undermine a client's life or self-image. We look for inaccurate things our clients believe about themselves and about life at an emotional level, and then we work with them to shape that emotional conviction into an explicit statement of their old learning so that a juxtaposition experience can be set up.

Sandra's Story

Although fit and slim, Sandra had a lifelong struggle with sweets, alternating between binges and total abstinence. In a session devoted to this issue, Sandra declared, "I just can't control myself. I've never shown any ability to control myself. I don't believe it's *possible* for me to stop eating sweets." This was a deep-seated emotional "truth" about eating that had wormed its way into her self-concept. Sandra felt helpless over sweets and afraid of her lack of control because her unconscious learning was that she was powerless to stop.

I encouraged her to repeat that belief out loud several times, with full conviction. Then I asked her if it was absolutely true, absolutely every time, that she couldn't control herself (Katie, 2002).

Sandra had proven her self-control through a lifetime of educational accomplishment, mature decisions, and a strong sense of ethical responsibility. Considering this, Sandra paused and said, "Well, I have controlled myself when I wanted to. So I guess it's not true that I can't control myself." She had made the first step, now there was homework to do.

Both "facts" about Sandra couldn't literally be true, so I asked her to practice the experiential exercise of just presenting herself with the erroneous statement as truth. In my adaptation of Ecker and Hulley's (2005–2019) suggestions, I had her write down on a note-card, "I can't control myself," and read it aloud to herself twice a day as absolute truth, while also remaining aware of herself as a person who had succeeded in life through many instances of self-control. ("Just state it out loud as an absolute truth about yourself, *while* remembering everything else you know about yourself, and see what your mind does with it.")

Alternatively, I could've asked her to write down both explicit beliefs ("I can't control myself" and "I have a good ability to control myself") and read them together, simultaneously presenting them both to her brain in split-screen fashion as real and true in order to set up the mismatch-and-error sensation. But I've found that simply saying the often ridiculous belief out loud *while* being in touch with current adult self-knowledge often seems equally effective in shifting the client's perception.

You might think such statements could be a dangerous form of negative self-affirmation, but people are more complex than that. We weren't programming a computer with malware; we were setting up an experience for Sandra's adult mind to reconsider an old belief in the larger context of who she knew herself to be. Sandra found that after a few rounds of spoken repetitions, her mind spontaneously balked at the old "truth" of being someone who can't control herself. Hearing herself affirm the old schema out loud bucked up against her common sense and self-knowledge, prompting her mind to spontaneously reject its emotional "truth." The outdated schema now seemed untrue and absurd. Her knowledge of reality resolved the contradiction in favor of the evidence that she *was* capable of controlling herself very well, not just around sweets but in her life in general.

Stated so plainly, Sandra's demoralizing belief bothered her mind into rejecting it as untrue, since it didn't fit reality. Because she had never before *consciously* held up the old emotional learning as incontestable truth, she never noticed that it didn't fit the facts of herself. To translate this into parts work, we could say we were having a child part of her state what it had learned, so her adult self could hear it as not true.

Although this may seem like CBT, it's significantly different. CBT might have counteracted Sandra's emotional learning ("I can't control myself") by thinking more realistic arguments for a different point of view. But by simply using the juxtaposition method, the client is not being explicitly told what or how to think. All they are being asked to do is to expose and state clearly the old learning they've assumed to be true, experientially juxtapose it against a more current belief, and then let the brain decide which reality is more accurate.

There's no hard work involved; you're just taking advantage of what the brain already does naturally, as long as the contradictory statements are presented to it in a clear enough fashion. Thank goodness for this natural brain hack; otherwise, human beings would have to sort through outdated mind clutter for every new problem, not to mention running out of room for new learning. The neuroplasticity of the brain overwrites or erases the feeling of "truth" as soon as it realizes that the old learning couldn't possibly still be correct. The brain then relegates the old memory-fact to the dead-letter file and busies itself in accommodating the new reality it now accepts (Ecker, 2015, 2024).

After Sandra's mind spontaneously reshaped her self-assessment to fit the more accurate reality, we further refined her understanding of the situation: it wasn't that she "couldn't control herself," but that she had trouble limiting her intake of sweets if she allowed herself to start gobbling them impulsively and compulsively for days on end. Notice that this was coming from our processing together, not from my explicitly assigning the correct cognition. I just asked the questions that helped her keep comparing these learnings.

Sandra now realized she *could* control herself if she observed certain limits. This shifted the low self-esteem that had bedeviled her over her supposed lack of control. It was unrealistic for her to think that self-control meant that she should be able to eat a binge-trigger food—a kind of addictive substance for her—any time she wanted and not feel any temptation to go further. Later, Sandra and I reshaped her self-belief statement into "I *can* control my sweet tooth *when* I stay aware of triggering foods and the onset of urges" as a new part of her self-concept. But at first she had to simultaneously *experience* the relative truth of these two beliefs—"I can't control myself" *and* "I do control myself"—before tackling any refinements or conditions.

Giving Up Old Realities May Spark Grief

Once the old learning is dismantled and updated through memory reconsolidation, your client may feel grief and regret as they realize that the old emotional learning behind their symptoms and suffering was based on an erroneous conclusion. Many times, a client doesn't know how constrained they were by old mental models until they're gone. Then there can be anger or sorrow over what they've been deprived of as a result.

At such a point, you can engage your client in the meta-therapeutic processing that we discussed in chapter 9 (*What was that like for you to talk with me about that? How did it feel to experience with me that the old learning wasn't true?*). Sometimes asking them how they felt doing the juxtapositions with you can open up these regretful feelings, and also build emotional intimacy between you and your client.

To be sure that transformational change has occurred, Ecker and Hulley (2005–2019) encourage therapists to check back later to confirm that the schema has lost its emotional realness, is no longer triggered by certain signals, and no longer fuels symptoms. If the therapy has worked, staying free from old schemas should be mostly effortless.

Appendices

Personality Characteristics of Emotionally Immature People

Personality Structure

- Rigid and simplistic; not complex inside; tend to alter scary reality by narrowing it down

- Poor self-development, characterized by many disconnected and/or poorly integrated parts

- All-or-nothing emotions, experiencing everything as black and white, good or bad

- Inconsistent and contradictory beliefs and actions, characteristic of a lack of personality integration

Attitude Toward Reality

- Driven to deny, distort, or dismiss reality when it causes them tension

- Self-referential, but not self-reflective; all roads lead to them; show no self-doubt

- Focus is on physical, material aspects of the world and other people, to the exclusion of the emotional or psychological

Emotional Characteristics

- Intense but shallow emotions

- Show affective realism (Barrett & Bar, 2009): "Reality is what it *feels* like to me"

- Do more reacting than thinking; do what feels best and relieves tension

- No mixed feelings, little modulation or nuance of emotion

Defenses and Coping Mechanisms

- Egocentric, self-preoccupied, can't stop thinking about themselves

- Low stress tolerance, impatient, closed-minded, one-track mind

- Strongly defensive and critical of the unfamiliar

- Poor self-observation, can't think objectively about their own thinking or behavior; not self-reflective

- Tend toward concrete, literal thinking, *or* obsessive intellectualizing

- Lack of continuity of time leading to poor accountability: "That was then, this is now"

- Immature defenses (Vaillant, G. E., 2000)

Interpersonal

- Low empathy, insensitive, often provoke anger and frustration in others

- Subjective, not objective; rejects other points of view, uncomfortable with differences

- Use emotional coercion (shame, guilt, fear, self-doubt) and emotional takeovers

- Do not do emotional work; limited capacity for relationship repair

- Enmeshment or superficiality instead of emotional intimacy

- Killjoy responses to others' happiness: tend toward sadism, meanness, contempt, envy, mockery, sarcasm, cynicism

- Poor direct communication: use emotional contagion, projective identification

- Terrified of deep emotion and emotional intimacy

- Hard to give to (poor receptive capacity (Vaillant, L. M., 1997)

- Require mirroring, praise, admiration, specialness, authority

- Demand role reversals: others should care for them under all circumstances

- Roles are sacred: role entitlement, role coercion, caretaker role-reversal

- Play favorites, seeking people to enmesh with

Appendix B

Emotional Immaturity and Emotional Maturity Compared

Emotional Immaturity	Emotional Maturity
Thoughts about life are simplistic, literal, and rigid. Dislike the uncertainty of an evolving reality.	Appreciate the nuances of life and how things are constantly changing.
A need to control others through guilt, anger, or shame.	Aware they cannot and do not want to control others.
View others as incompetent.	See shortcomings as a part of being human.
Express charm and charisma.	Express warmth and sincerity.
Define self and others by their roles in a binary way: submissive or dominant.	Equitable view of all humans and comfortable without a social ranking system in place.
Poor filters; say whatever comes to mind without regard for others' feelings. Claim it is "being honest."	Share feelings from their own experience in mutually respectful ways.
Poor listeners, unattuned, and unable to resonate with others who disagree with them.	Deep listeners, meaning-focused, able to attune to self and others.
Resist and deny reality, especially when it does not fit with their opinions.	Integrate new information with acceptance even if it is uncomfortable.

Emotional Immaturity	*Emotional Maturity*
"Affective realism"—things are as they feel at the moment.	The facts do not change because you experience intense feelings.
Unable to learn from errors because actions are not connected as a possible cause of harm to others.	Can self-correct and grow, owning and learning from mistakes.
Fundamentally fearful and insecure.	Sense of self strong enough to self-regulate emotional safety.
Defend what is familiar because complexity is overwhelming.	Open to changing their minds when new information comes to light.
Do not trust or desire to learn or comprehend complex concepts.	Enjoy learning even if it contradicts what they already believe.
Rigid about rules but change the rules when it benefits them.	Place people before rules, live in grace, can identify ideology and dogma.
Proud of being unyielding and judgmental but call their rigid thinking "moral fortitude."	Flexibility in thinking patterns. Able to update opinions based on new information.
Use superficial logic to shut down other people's feelings. "You shouldn't feel that way because…"	Accept that others feel what they feel.
Believe that if only others would plan well enough, they can avoid all mistakes, and others should always feel bad about their mistakes.	Believe that mistakes are a normal part of life. Able to own mistakes and make sincere repair attempts for healing and growth.
See other people's boundaries as something to overcome.	See other people's boundaries as healthy and something to respect.
Dismiss or scoff at personal growth. Are threatened by the suggestion they are not perfect.	Enjoy the journey of personal growth. Aware they are imperfect and loveable.

Appendix C

Bill of Rights for Adult Children of Emotionally Immature Parents

1. The Right to Set Limits

- ☐ I have the right to set limits on your hurtful or exploitative behavior.
- ☐ I have the right to break off any interaction in which I feel pressured or coerced.
- ☐ I have the right to stop anything long before I feel exhausted.
- ☐ I have the right to call a halt to any interaction I don't find enjoyable.
- ☐ I have the right to say no without a good reason.

2. The Right Not to be Emotionally Coerced

- ☐ I have the right to not be your rescuer.
- ☐ I have the right to ask you to get help from someone else.
- ☐ I have the right to not fix your problems.
- ☐ I have the right to let you manage your own self-esteem without my input.
- ☐ I have the right to let you handle your own distress.
- ☐ I have the right to refuse to feel guilty.

3. The Right to Emotional Autonomy and Mental Freedom

- ☐ I have the right to any and all of my feelings.

- ☐ I have the right to think anything I want.

- ☐ I have the right to not be ridiculed or mocked about my values, ideas, or interests.

- ☐ I have the right to be bothered by how I'm treated.

- ☐ I have the right to not like your behavior or attitude.

4. The Right to Choose Relationships

- ☐ I have the right to know whether I love you or not.

- ☐ I have the right to refuse what you want to give me.

- ☐ I have the right not to be disloyal to myself just to make things easier on you.

- ☐ I have the right to end our relationship, even if we're related.

- ☐ I have the right not to be depended upon.

- ☐ I have the right to stay away from anyone who is unpleasant or draining.

5. The Right to Clear Communications

- ☐ I have the right to say anything as long as I do so in a nonviolent, nonharmful way.

- ☐ I have the right to ask to be listened to.

- ☐ I have the right to tell you my feelings are hurt.

- ☐ I have the right to speak up and tell you what I really prefer.

- ☐ I have the right to be told what you want from me without assuming I should know.

6. The Right to Choose What's Best for Me

☐ I have the right not to do things if it's not a good time for me.

☐ I have the right to leave whenever I want.

☐ I have the right to say no to activities or get-togethers I don't find enjoyable.

☐ I have the right to make my own decisions, without self-doubt.

7. The Right to Live Life My Own Way

☐ I have the right to take action even if you don't think it's a good idea.

☐ I have the right to spend my energy and time on what I find important.

☐ I have the right to trust my inner experiences and take my aspirations seriously.

☐ I have the right to take all the time I need and not be rushed.

8. The Right to Equal Importance and Respect

☐ I have the right to be considered just as important as you.

☐ I have the right to live my life without ridicule from anyone.

☐ I have the right to be treated respectfully as an independent adult.

☐ I have the right to refuse to feel shame.

9. The Right to Put My Own Health and Well-Being First

☐ I have the right to thrive, not just survive.

☐ I have the right to take time for myself to do what I enjoy.

☐ I have the right to decide how much energy and attention I give to other people.

☐ I have the right to take time to think things over.

☐ I have the right to take care of myself regardless of what others think.

☐ I have the right to take the time and space necessary to nourish my inner world.

10. The Right to Love and Protect Myself

☐ I have the right to self-compassion when I make mistakes.

☐ I have the right to change my self-concept when it no longer fits.

☐ I have the right to love myself and treat myself nicely.

☐ I have the right to be free of self-criticism and to enjoy my individuality.

☐ I have the right to be me.

Appendix D

The EIP Unspoken Relationship Contract

To remain in good standing with an emotionally immature person, I consent to the following:

1. I agree that your needs should come before anyone else's.

2. I agree not to speak my own mind when I'm around you.

3. Please say anything you want, and I won't object.

4. Yes, I must be ignorant if I think differently from you.

5. Of course you should be upset if anyone says no to you about anything.

6. Please educate me about what I should like or dislike.

7. Yes, it makes sense for you to decide how much time I should want to spend with you.

8. You're right, I should show you "respect" by disowning my own thoughts in your presence.

9. Of course you shouldn't have to exercise self-control if you don't feel like it.

10. It's fine if you don't think before you speak.

11. It's true: you should never have to wait or deal with any unpleasantness.

12. I agree, you shouldn't have to adjust when circumstances change around you.

13. It's okay if you ignore me, snap at me, or don't act glad to see me. I'll still want to spend time with you.

14. Of course you are entitled to be rude.

15. I agree that you shouldn't have to take directions from anyone.

16. Please talk as long as you like about your favorite topics; I'm ready to just listen and never be asked any questions about myself.

Reprinted from Gibson, L. C., 2019, *Recovering from Emotionally Immature Parents*, pp. 178–179. Oakland, CA: New Harbinger Publications.

Self-Concept Quiz

You can ask your client to answer the following question and complete the statements to get at how they were trained to think about themselves.

- What was your role in the family?

- I was the kid most likely to...

- I think my mother thought I was...

- My father saw me as...

- My best quality is my ability to...

- I am different from my family because I...

- I see myself as...

- What I most like about myself is...

- What I would most like to change about myself is...

- I need to be more...

Appendix F

Writing Therapy: A Brief Guide on Using Writing to Get Unstuck*

Q: When should I do this?

A: When you feel overwhelmed and stuck! Putting the contents of your mind down on paper should be in every home's first aid manual. It's the single most effective self-help method you can use when circumstances have outrun your ability to keep up. When you are getting nowhere with your actions, it may be because you don't know what is *really* upsetting you.

Q: Why should I do this?

A: To figure out what triggered you and to avoid creating even more chaos! When you take action before you know your true feelings, your blind reactions may create mayhem around you. Now you have a second problem to deal with caused by reacting impulsively to the first problem.

Q: How should I use this?

- Instead of reacting impulsively or dissociating (like numbing out, scrolling on your phone, etc.), sit down with a piece of paper and pen and write **without** self-censoring.

---

* Adapted from Gibson, L. C., 2021, *Self-Care for Adult Children of Emotionally Immature Parents.* Oakland, CA: New Harbinger Publications.

References

Karpman, S. 1968. Fairy tales and script drama analysis. *Transactional Analysis Bulletin*, *26*(7), 39–43.

Katie, B. 2002. *Loving What Is*. New York: Three Rivers Press.

Krystal, H. 1988/2009. *Integration and Self-Healing*. New York: Routledge.

Langs, R. 1978. *The Listening Process*. New York: Jason Aronson.

Levine, P. 1997. *Waking the Tiger*. Berkeley, CA: North Atlantic Books.

———. 2005/2008. *Healing Trauma*. Boulder, CO: Sounds True.

Levinson, D. J. 1978. *The Seasons of a Man's Life*. New York: Ballentine Books.

Lewis, T., Amini, F., & Lannon, R. 2000. *A General Theory of Love*. New York: Vintage Books.

Mahler, M., Pine, F., & Bergman, A. 1975. *The Psychological Birth of the Human Infant*. New York: Basic Books.

Marlow-MaCoy, A. 2020. *The Gaslighting Recovery Workbook*. Emeryville, CA: Rockridge Press.

Maier, S. F., & Seligman, M. E. P. 2016. Learned helplessness at fifty: Insights from neuroscience. *Psychological Review*, *123*(4), 349–367. https://doi.org/10.1037/rev0000033

Maté, G. 2003. *When the Body Says No*. Hoboken, NJ: John Wiley & Sons.

McCullough, L., Kuhn, N., Andrews, S., Kaplan, A., Wolf, J., & Hurley, C. 2003. *Treating Affect Phobia*. New York: Guilford Press.

McGilchrist, I. 2009. *The Master and His Emissary*. New Haven, CT: Yale University Press.

———. 2013. Hemisphere differences and their relevance to psychotherapy. In D. J. Siegel and M. Solomon (Eds.), *Healing Moments in Psychotherapy* (pp. 67–88). New York: W. W. Norton.

———. 2021. *The Matter with Things, Vol I & II*. London: Perspectiva Press.

Mendaglio, S. (Ed.). 2008. *Dabrowski's Theory of Positive Disintegration*. Scottsdale, AZ: Great Potential Press.

Miller, A. 1981. *The Drama of the Gifted Child*. New York: Basic Books.

———. 1997. *The Essential Role of an Enlightened Witness in Society*. https://www.alice-miller.com/en/the-essential-role-of-an-enlightened-witness-in-society

Minuchin, S. 1974. *Families and Family Therapy*. Cambridge, MA: Harvard University Press.

Minuchin, S., Montalvo, B., Guerney, B. G., Rosman, B. L., & Schumer, F. 1967. *Families of the Slums*. New York: Basic Books.

Ogden, T. H. 1982. *Projective Identification and Psychoanalytic Technique*. Northvale, NJ: Jason Aronson.

Ogrodniczuk, J. S., Piper, W. E., & Joyce, A. S. 2011. Effect of Alexithymia on the process and outcome of psychotherapy: a programmatic review. *Psychiatry Research, 190*(1), 43–48.

Patterson, K., Grenny, J., McMillan, R., & Switzler, A. 2012. *Crucial Conversations.* New York: McGraw-Hill.

Pennebaker, J. W., & Beall, S. K. 1986. Confronting a traumatic event: toward an understanding of inhibition and disease. *Journal of Abnormal Psychology, 95*(3), 274–281.

Perera, A. 2023. Implicit and explicit memory: definition and examples. *Simply Psychology.* https://www.simplypsychology.org/implicit-versus-explicit-memory.html

Perls, F. 1969/1992. *Gestalt Therapy Verbatim.* Gouldsboro, ME: The Gestalt Journal Press.

Piaget, J. 1963. *The Psychology of Intelligence.* New York: Littlefield, Adams.

Porges, S. 2011. *The Polyvagal Theory: Neurophysiological Foundations of Emotions, Attachment, Communication, Self-Regulation.* New York: W. W. Norton.

———. 2017. *The Pocket Guide to the Polyvagal Theory.* New York: W. W. Norton.

Porges, S., & Porges, S. 2023. *Our Polyvagal World.* New York: W. W. Norton.

Premack, D., & Woodruff, G. 1978. Does the chimpanzee have a theory of mind? *Behavioral and Brain Sciences, 1*(4), 515–526. https://doi.org/10.1017/S0140525X00076512

Puder, D. 2019. The problem of disconnection: the still face experiment. *Psychiatry and Psychotherapy* YouTube channel. https://www.youtube.com/watch?v=HnhOG76 WaFc&t=3s

Rizzolatti, G. 2005. The mirror neuron system and its function in humans. *Anatomy and Embryology, 210,* 419–421. https://doi.org/10.1007/s00429-005-0039-z

Rizzolatti, G., & Craighero, L. 2004. The mirror-neuron system. *Annual Review of Neuroscience, 27,* 169–192. 10.1146/annurev.neuro.27.070203.144230

Rogers, C. R. 1961/1989. *On Becoming a Person.* New York: Houghton Mifflin Company.

———. 1980. *A Way of Being.* New York: HarperCollins Publishers.

Rosenberg, M. 2015. *Nonviolent Communication.* Encinitas, CA: Puddle-Dancer Press.

Rotter, J. B., Lah, M. I., & Rafferty, J. E. 1992. *Rotter Incomplete Sentences Blank.* San Antonio, TX: Harcourt Brace.

Rotter, J. B., & Willerman, B. 1947. The Incomplete Sentences Test as a method of studying personality. *Journal of Consulting Psychology, 11,* 43–48.

Ruf, D. 2023. *The 5 Levels of Gifted Children Grown Up.* Golden Valley, MN: 5LoG Press.

Sapolsky, R. M. 1994/1998. *Why Zebras Don't Get Ulcers.* New York: Barnes & Noble/W. H. Freeman.

Schacter, D. L. 1987. Implicit memory: History and current status. *Journal of Experimental Psychology: Learning, Memory, and Cognition, 13*(3), 501–518.

Schore, A. 2009. Right brain affect regulation: An essential mechanism of development, trauma, dissociation, and psychotherapy. In D. Fosha, D. J. Siegel & M. F. Soloman (Eds.), *The Healing Power of Emotion* (pp. 112–144). New York: W. W. Norton.

Schore, A. 2012. *The Science of the Art of Psychotherapy.* New York: W. W. Norton.

———. 2019. *Right Brain Psychotherapy.* New York: W. W. Norton.

———. 2022. Right brain-to-right brain psychotherapy: recent scientific and clinical advances. *Annals of General Psychiatry, 21,* 46. https://doi.org/10.1186/s12991-022-00420-3

Schwartz, R. 1995. *Internal Family Systems.* New York: Guilford Press.

———. 2001. *Introduction to the Internal Family Systems Model.* Oak Park, IL: Trailheads Publications.

———. 2021. *No Bad Parts.* Boulder, CO: Sounds True.

Shaw, D. 2014. *Traumatic Narcissism.* New York: Routledge.

Sheehy, G. 1995. *New Passages.* New York: Ballentine Books.

Siegel, D. J. 2010a. *Mindsight.* New York: Bantam Books.

———. 2010b. *The Mindful Therapist.* New York: W. W. Norton.

Siegel, R. D. 2010. *The Mindfulness Solution.* New York: Guilford Press.

Seligman, M. E. P. 1972. Learned helplessness. *Annual Review of Medicine, 23*(1), 407–412. https://doi.org/10.1146/annurev.me.23.020172.002203

Southwick, S. M., & Charney, D. S. 2018. *Resilience.* Oxford: Cambridge University Press.

Spengler, P. M., Lee, N. A., & Wittenborn, A. K. 2022. A comprehensive meta-analysis on the efficacy of emotionally focused couple therapy. *Couple and Family Psychology: Research and Practice.* Advance online publication. http://doi.org/10.1037/cfp0000233

Stefano, A. 2015. The origins of the notion of countertransference. *The Psychoanalytic Review, 102*(4), 437–60. https://doi.org/10.1521/prev.2015.102.4.437

Stern, D. 1985. *The Interpersonal World of the Infant.* New York: Basic Books.

Stone, D., Patton, B., & Heen, S. 1999. *Difficult Conversations.* New York: Penguin Group.

Tawwab, N. G. 2021. *Set Boundaries, Find Peace.* New York: TarcherPerigee.

Taylor, K. 2004. *Brainwashing.* New York: Oxford University Press.

Taylor, J. B. 2021. *Whole Brain Living.* Carlsbad, CA: Hay House.

Terr, L. 1990. *Too Scared to Cry.* New York: Basic Books.

Tronick, E. 2007. *The Neurobehavioral and Social-Emotional Development of Infants and Children.* New York: W. W. Norton.

Trudeau, G. 2023. The best PTSD treatment you've never heard of. *The Washington Post.* https://www.washingtonpost.com/opinions/2023/07/10/ptsd-treatment-veterans -medicine-mental-health

Truman, K. 1991/2003. *Feelings Buried Alive Never Die.* St. George, UT: Olympic Distributing.

Tweedy, R. 2021. *The Divided Therapist.* New York: Routledge.

United Nations. 1948. *Universal Declaration of Human Rights.* http://www.un.org/en /universal-declaration-human-rights

Vaillant, G. E. 1977. *Adaptation to Life.* Cambridge, MA: Harvard University Press.

———. 1993. *The Wisdom of the Ego.* Cambridge, MA: Harvard University Press.

———. 2000. Adaptive mental mechanisms: their role in a positive psychology. *American Psychologist, 55,* 89–98.

Vaillant, L. M. 1997. *Changing Character.* New York: Basic Books.

van der Kolk, B. 2014. *The Body Keeps the Score.* New York: Viking Penguin.

Wallace, J. B. 2023. *Never Enough.* New York: Portfolio/Penguin.

Wallin, D. J. 2007/2015. *Attachment in Psychotherapy.* New York: Guilford Press.

Wampold, B. E. 2015. How important are the common factors in psychotherapy? An update. *World Psychiatry, 14,* 270–277.

Werner, E. E. 1993. Risk, resilience, and recovery: Perspectives from the Kauai Longitudinal Study. *Development and Psychopathology, 5*(4), 503–515. https://doi.org/10.1017/S0954 57940000612X

Werner, E. E., & Smith, R. S. 1992. *Overcoming the Odds: High Risk Children from Birth to Adulthood.* Ithaca, NY: Cornell University Press.

White, M. 2007. *Maps of Narrative Practice.* New York: W. W. Norton.

Winnicott, D. W. 1965/2018. *The Maturational Processes and the Facilitating Environment.* New York: Routledge.

———. 1989/2018. *Psychoanalytic Explorations.* New York: Routledge.

———. 2002. *Winnicott on the Child.* New York: Perseus Publishing.

Wolynn, M. 2016. *It Didn't Start with You.* New York: Penguin Random House.

Young, J., Klosko, J., & Weishaar, M. 2003. *Schema Therapy.* New York: Guilford Press.

Lindsay C. Gibson, PsyD, is a clinical psychologist and psychotherapist with more than thirty years' experience working in public service and private practice. Her books—including the *New York Times* bestseller, *Adult Children of Emotionally Immature Parents*—have sold more than a million copies, and have been translated into thirty-seven languages. In the past, Gibson has served as an adjunct assistant professor, teaching doctoral clinical psychology students clinical theory and psychotherapy techniques. She specializes in therapy and coaching with adults to attain new levels of personal growth, emotional intimacy with others, and confidence in dealing with emotionally immature family members. Gibson lives and works in Virginia Beach, VA.

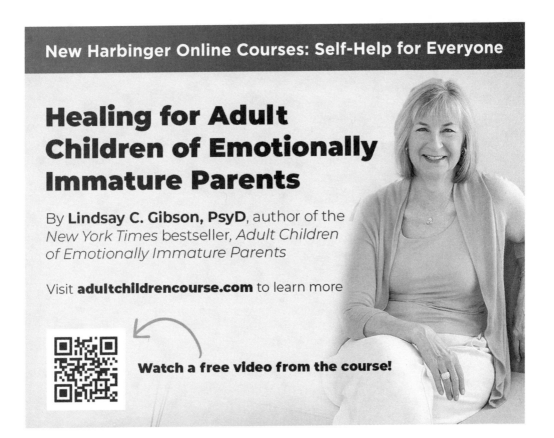

Index

Did you know there are **free tools** you can download for this book?

Free tools are things like **worksheets**, **guided meditation exercises**, and **more** that will help you get the most out of your book.

You can download free tools for this book—whether you bought or borrowed it, in any format, from any source—from the New Harbinger website. All you need is a NewHarbinger.com account. Just use the URL provided in this book to view the free tools that are available for it. Then, click on the "download" button for the free tool you want, and follow the prompts that appear to log in to your NewHarbinger.com account and download the material.

You can also save the free tools for this book to your **Free Tools Library** so you can access them again anytime, just by logging in to your account! Just look for this button on the book's free tools page.

+ Save this to my free tools library

If you need help accessing or downloading free tools, visit **newharbinger.com/faq** or contact us at **customerservice@newharbinger.com**.